The Thriving Vegan

Vegan

How to Discover the Foods Your Body Loves

MICHAEL J. DORFMAN

ISBN-13: 9781095677667

Dedicated to my wife and life partner Delia. Since 2010, she has inspired me with her whole food vegan cooking, convincing me that anyone who likes to cook, and is interested in achieving optimal health, can create amazing and simple meals, with plant based foods.

TABLE OF CONTENTS

2   Our Body's Healing Powers

3   Refuting The Sacred Cows of Nutrition

4   Doctors, Drugs and The Medical Profession

5 Are We Being Duped?

6 Health: Personal, Animal and The Planet

Recommended Resources   212

INTRODUCTION

WHY I CHANGED TO WHOLE PLANT BASED (VEGAN) FOODS

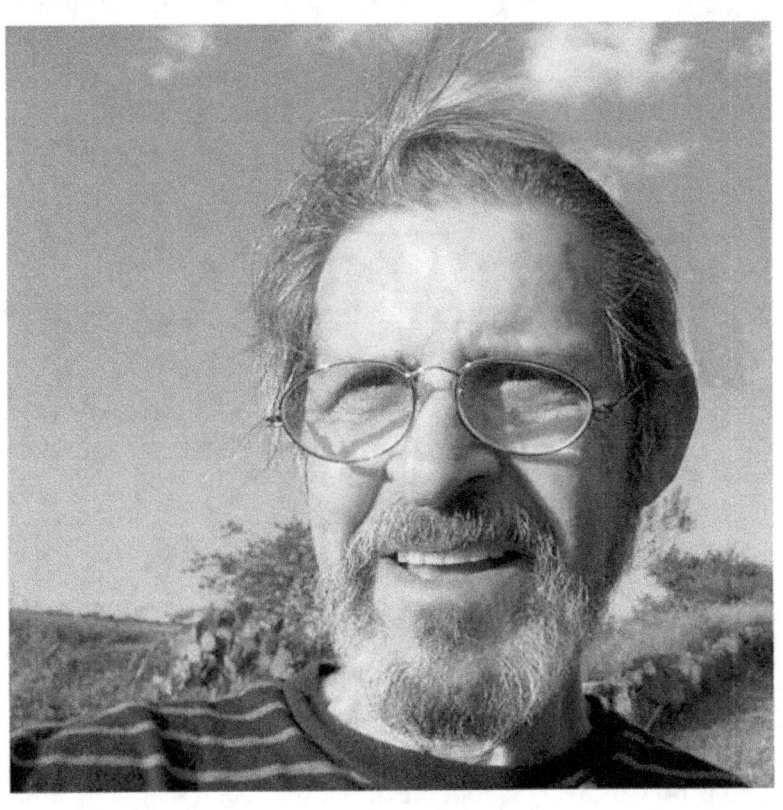

It was during the 1970's, when I first became attracted to Zen philosophy, that I became a vegetarian. Not consuming meat has always been an integral part of certain Eastern civilizations. Until that time, like most Americans, I was eating the Standard American Diet (SAD) of meat, dairy, eggs, lots of processed foods and some fruits and vegetables. In my family there were several butchers, including my father, my brother, two uncles and a cousin so, as you could well imagine, we ate lots of meat...at least once a day. I never questioned whether so much meat was healthy and just like most people, during the 1950's, I just ate what my mother put in front of me. It didn't matter whether it was steak, cow or chicken livers, pancreas, bellybutton, tongue or even brains. So, on this one special day, in 1976, I gave up eating all meats (and stopped smoking too!). I also started reading books on nutrition and health and discovered that that there were doctors and health care professionals who were actually reversing heart disease by simply changing a person's diet...to whole plant based foods. Although I became interested in this new approach, I found it extremely difficult to give up consuming dairy products... especially cheese (loved that pizza!).

However, as time went by, I became somewhat concerned about my health because I would become ill 2 or 3 times a year...with a cough, sore throat and chest and nasal congestion. Although not life threatening, they weren't very pleasant experiences, to say the least. In 2010, my brother Arthur, who is now in his 80s, told me about his vegan diet, which he had been following for more than 20 years. He believed that it could be the dairy that was causing the congestion and the other symptoms I was experiencing. He suggested that I give veganism a try...so I did...and the rest is history. Since making the change, those annual illnesses are now only a memory...a thing of the past.

The story of Beatriz

The inspiration to pass on to others what I have been experiencing and learning, during these past years, started with my friend Beatriz from Cozumel, Mexico, who underwent quadruple bypass surgery in 2011. Although she survived the operation, a year later she began suffering from recurring pain in her arm. After an examination and tests she was told that a stent would be required to open up the newly clogged artery. Unfortunately, the stent didn't fit, so the surgeon told her that there was nothing more to do. To accept this conclusion would be to accept that her life was pretty much over at age 72. What they didn't tell her, but told my wife and her son, was that she had about 6 months to live. Looking back now, I believe it was fortunate that she didn't know. When doctors tell a patient how long he or she has left, more often than not, depression sets in and all hope evaporates.

I spoke to her about Whole Food Vegan Nutrition and after concluding that there were not many alternatives available, Beatriz decided to give it a try. I also gave her a copy of Dr. Caldwell Esselstyn's book "Prevent and Reverse Heart Disease. Within weeks her health began to improve and today, seven years later, she is alive and kicking in Cozumel. Although the doctors had given up hope, for me her recovery has been near miraculous. As soon as she stopped eating the artery-clogging foods that contributed to her heart disease, her body started to heal itself.

With this Startling Result I Began to Ask Myself some Intriguing Questions:

A   If heart disease is the number one global killer why wasn't food being considered as the go to preventive diet as well as an integral part of heart disease therapy?

B   Why don't doctor's inform their patients about the importance of nutrition following bypass surgery?

C   If nutrition can be such an important factor in reversing heart disease, are there other chronic diseases that can be reversed as well?

TO ANSWER THESE AND OTHER QUESTIONS ABOUT THE CONNECTION BETWEEN HEALTH AND NUTRITION, IN A CLEAR AND SENSIBLE WAY, IS THE MAIN OBJECTIVE OF THIS BOOK.

For those of us who grew up eating the Standard American Diet (SAD), starting to eat healthfully can be a big shift — I know it was for me. Now, in 2019 and at the age of 77 I am completely committed to Whole Food Vegan Nutrition and, as a result, have so far been able to escape SAD's clutches. Looking back, I view that as one of the best decisions of my life. Eating healthier is easier than you think, it's inexpensive, and it just might save your life.

THE "YEAR OF THE VEGAN"...AND BEYOND

The Guardian calls 2019 "The Year of the Vegan"

Maclean's—one of Canada's oldest magazines—has declared 2019 "The Year of the Vegan"

The Economist's "The World in 2019" predicts that veganism will be the most popular topic of the new year, declaring 2019 "The Year Veganism Goes Mainstream."

Forbes published an article predicting that 2019 will be the year more people "Embrace a Plant-Based Lifestyle."

10 Reasons Why 2019 Will Be a Pivotal Year in Determining What Foods Human Beings Will Be Consuming in the Future:

1 Decades of research and studies are proving that plant based foods can prevent and reverse severe illnesses and chronic diseases.

2 Doctors and Health Care Professionals are offering <u>free</u> online plant based conferences and forums covering various health topics.

3 Online documentaries (i.e. Netflix) are exposing the global horrors of animal exploitation on factory farms.

4 Besides the negative effects that automobiles and industry are having on world climate, scientific studies are now providing evidence that shows the impact that factory farms are having on the environment, including the contamination and reduction of global water supplies and available arable land.

5 In the United States, institutions such as The American Medical Association, American Heart Association and

the American Cancer Society have been emphasizing the need to consume more plant based foods in order to avoid chronic diseases.

6 "Big Meat" businesses are investing in plant based foods. Tyson, America's largest meat producer, invested in the vegan company, Beyond Meat. Canada's major meat company Maple Leaf Foods has launched an independent subsidiary called Greenleaf Foods that is 100% plant based. Applegate Farms, a subsidiary of meat giant Hormel Foods (Herdez, Skippy, Del Fuerte, Búfalo, Doña María) aims to invest in the $3.7 billion plant-based market. In Chicago, McDonald's now offers the Vegan Burger and Domino's Australia, having heard the opinions of the people, will now offer dairy-free cheese pizzas at over 600 locations nationwide. Ice cream giants, Baskin and Robbins and Ben and Jerry's are now offering dairy free ice cream and Dean Foods Company, the largest dairy producer in the United States known for its DairyPure brand, has invested in the plant-based milk and yogurt company Good Karma Foods. Danone, recently completed it's purchase of WhiteWave Foods, producer of dairy-free brands such as So Delicious, Silk, and Vega. Maybe these moves by major companies are not because of their interest in our health, but more like an interest in their "bottom line." Whatever the reason, it's a step in the right direction.

7 Elite professional and amateur athletes, from a variety of sports (football, soccer, basketball, tennis,

basketball, boxing, martial arts, bodybuilders, etc.) are attesting to improved performances and improved health and wellbeing, when they switched to plant based foods.

8 The availability of thousands of simple, as well as gourmet, vegan recipes in health books and on the internet.

9 With the prediction of a global population of 10 billion by 2050, and because of the growing need for freshwater and arable land in order to produce enough meat, dairy and eggs to meet the demand…it is becoming clear that the present trend is not sustainable.

10 On our present course, scientists are predicting catastrophic consequences to the planet and all living creatures…during the next 20 years.

The Four Main Reasons why people become vegans:

A Personal interest in living a long and healthy life, free from common illnesses and the pain and suffering from chronic diseases.

B Interest in stopping and reversing the growing world tendency towards catastrophic disease pandemics such as heart disease, cancer and type 2 Diabetes.

C Anger and Frustration because of the Exploitation of Animals, especially on factory farms.

D Belief that climate change is real and that human beings are guilty for much of Earth's devastation through the destruction of tropical forests and the mismanagement of land and water supplies.

What's the Solution?

My point of view:

"Since human beings are guilty of creating many of the global problems, they now face, they also have the capability of finding the solutions. And, as we shall see throughout this book, the main solution to A, B, C and D... can be found on our plates. All we need to do is make the connection."

On a personal level, although I am involved with reasons A, B, C and D, my primary interest is with A: <u>One's own Personal Health and Wellbeing</u>. Why? Because, from my perspective, in order to truly help other people, other species, or the planet, we should first help and take care of ourselves.

"THE THRIVING VEGAN" IS ABOUT UNLEARNING AND REDISCOVERING

Discovering the foods your body loves requires letting go of some of the concepts and ideas we've learned about nutrition, since we were very young...from our parents, our teachers, the media and even our doctors and health care providers. It's also about returning to the way that nature meant us to eat, as a species, just as nature has chosen specific foods for other species. Our pet cats and dogs know what foods are right for them, as do lions and tigers and bears...and elephants, cows, crocodiles, etc. There is no doubt. They are not confused...like we are. They don't have countless diets to choose from. The question is, as a species, shouldn't human beings also know what is right for them...for taste and for health reasons? I believe so. The problem is, that we don't know that we know and, as a result, we end up being prey to all the nutrition information and fads that are out there. We become confused…not knowing who or what to believe. Do these so called nutrition "experts" really care about our wellbeing or are they in it mainly for profit? Through unlearning and rediscovering the fundamentals of optimal nutrition I hope to shine a light on the situation, so that things will begin to make sense, and when something makes sense it becomes more meaningful than just more information. There is an understanding that takes place…a moment, a snap of the fingers, a nod of the head…when I could say to myself, yes, That Makes Sense!!

OUR BODY IS WHERE THE GIFT OF LIFE RESIDES

I have always felt that our greatest gift is the gift of life. Yes, we have the gifts of sight and hearing, the ability to think and imagine and to feel joy and love, among other things. But, none of this would be possible if we hadn't first received the gift of life.

However, I'd like to call your attention to another gift, which we don't often perceive as a gift and, as a result, take it for granted. It is this container or vessel… called the body. It is only through our body that we can experience the gift of life. Without it, life for you and me could not happen. That is the truth. The question is: If we truly accept and understand that our body is a gift and is our life's only home, shouldn't we do our utmost to respect it and take care of it, so that our experience of this "once in a lifetime" life becomes a wonderful and enjoyable journey?

On the contrary, if we do not accept it and understand it's preciousness, taking proper care of our body will not be that important. Instead, it will take it's place at the bottom of our list of our priorities...below making money, having a career, getting an education, buying a car, etc. As a result and as the years pass by, we may find ourselves a victim of the pain and suffering from illness and chronic diseases that can surely make the journey of life...a nightmare.

1

KNOWING LEADS TO CONSCIOUS CHOICES

The word is knowing - not belief - knowing.
How do you know? How do you know anything?
You have to be conscious to know, and you have to be
unconscious to not know.

— *Prem Rawat*

NOT ALL VEGANS ARE CREATED EQUAL
"Not all Vegans are Created Equal" simply means that following a vegan diet doesn't guarantee that it's a healthy diet, it just signifies that you're not consuming animal products. If you eat processed and refined foods, like sugars, white flours and white rice, you're not eating much healthier than someone on the Standard American Diet (SAD) of meat, dairy, eggs and refined and processed foods. In other words, you can eat only potato chips and donuts and drink coca cola every day and

rightfully call yourself a vegan but, how healthy is that? What I'm emphasizing here is Whole Food Vegan or Whole Food Plant Based nutrition, where the word "Whole" is key. The more processed foods are the greater the odds are for illness and chronic disease, somewhere down the line. So, if you know of someone who claims to be vegan but does not appear particularly healthy it could be because the quality of the food is not really his or her priority.

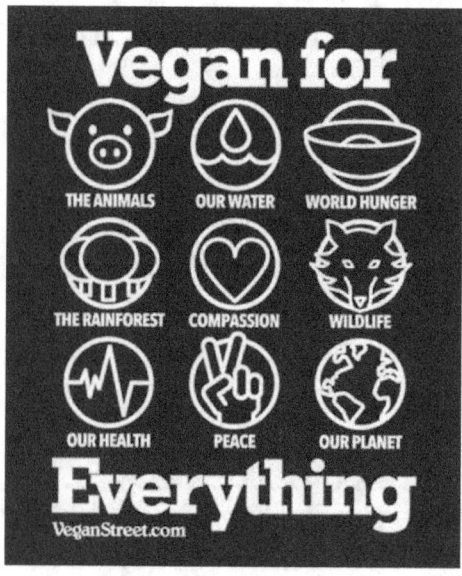

WHY IS THIS SO? Because people become vegans for different reasons:

1. For Personal Health and Wellbeing
2. Against Animal Exploitation and Cruelty
3. Survival of the Planet (Climate Change).

In other words, if a "vegan's" interest is mainly on 2 and 3, chances are that he or she may be compromising their health. In my opinion, since all 3 reasons are extremely important, for the survival of all species (including human beings) and the planet, the focus should be on all three.

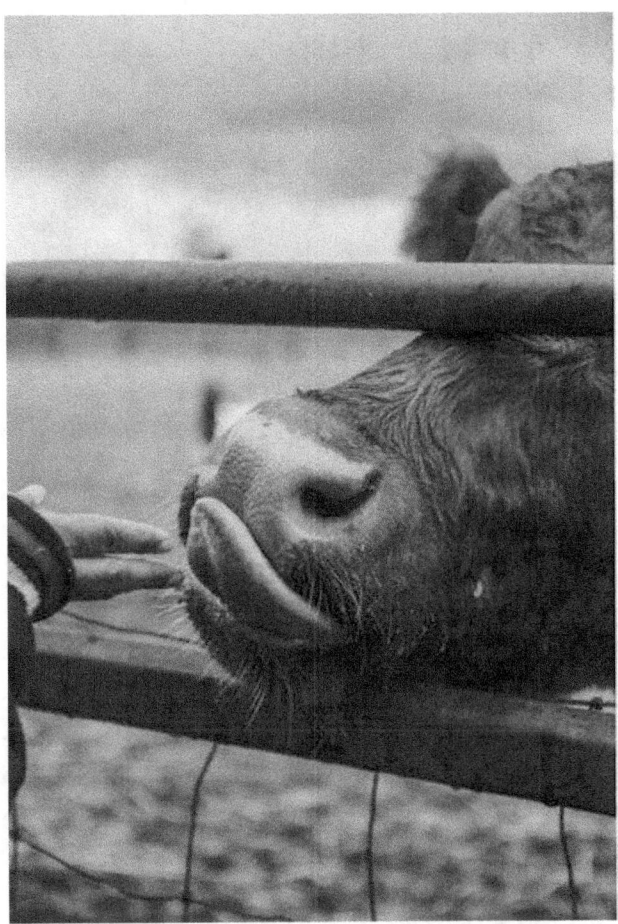

THE OMNIVORE DILEMMA

Throughout history we see that human beings have been nourished by animal products as well as by plants. Although I've searched high and low and left and right I've found "believable" arguments on both sides, to try to answer the question

— Are we omnivores or herbivores? If a person consumes meat, he or she can defend that choice by simply citing that stone age man ate meat. On the other hand, people who are vegetarians or vegans can claim that we are biologically connected to the plant eating great apes, including chimpanzees, gorillas, urangutans, etc. Some "humans" may not like the idea but the scientifically accepted Theory of Evolution, by Charles Darwin, explains that it is so.

When the Stone Age arrived it allowed man to make tools, including arrowheads and spears. As a result, we were capable of hunting and killing animals that were physically stronger and faster than we were. That led to a dilemma because, although we have pre-Stone Age coronary arteries and intestinal tracts, which evolved over millions of years…we were now consuming meat. According to an article in Psychology Today, The Truth About the Caveman Diet "The caveman diet is a great diet if you want to live to be 30 or 35 years old. That was the adult life expectancy until very, very recently (indeed, it wasn't until well after the advent of agriculture that life expectancy began to rise—in agricultural communities!). We know this from skeletal evidence. Individuals older than 40 at death are very rare in the Paleolithic record." The article goes on to say, "It wasn't that the caveman diet killed these people. It is just that almost no one lived long enough to develop the medical conditions we associate with long-term consumption of large quantities of animal protein and fat. Thus, just because cavemen did it does not mean it is good for you."

In other words, even if we agree that humans have been omnivores for a large part of their history, because they did not live long enough, we cannot automatically conclude that eating meat today is our healthiest choice. Furthermore, the meat we eat today, except for a few exceptions, is not the same as the meat that Paleo-man ate. Remember, he was a hunter... chasing after and killing wild game. The "game" was constantly on the move and "fit as a fiddle", in order to avoid being hunted down by man or any other predator. As a result, most animals were muscular with a very low body fat percentage. For example, a wild antelope generally has a Body Mass Index, which measures body fat, of 7%. Today, with the establishment of factory farms, cows carry 30% body fat (mostly saturated). For business...fat is good, because it "fattens" the wallet. Also, hormones and foods that fatten cows, chickens, pigs and goats, are replacing the foods that nature meant these animals to eat. Combine that with the ingestion of antibiotics, fed to these animals, for disease prevention, and it is clear that today's factory farm animals are a far cry from what our meat eating ancestors consumed.

So which is the healthiest choice ... today?

1) Populations that consume plant based foods are healthier and live longer than populations that are meat based. They include the 5 Blue Zone cultures, written about in the NY Times Best Seller, *"The Blue Zones"* and discovered by National Geographic explorer, Dan Buettner *(Okinawa, Japan, Loma Linda, California, Sardinia, Italy, Nicoya, Costa Rica and Nicaria, Greece). Other examples are populations living in the rural*

communities of China, Japan and parts of Africa. They have been thriving on plant based foods for centuries.

2) Populations that eat mostly animal based products (i.e., the Standard American Diet) continue to be at higher risk of chronic illnesses such as heart disease, cancer, type 2 diabetes, arthritis, osteoporosis, Alzheimer's, high blood pressure, etc.

3) More and more athletes are finding that changing from meat to plants has not only improved performance, but their health as well. They find that eating plant based foods **boosts blood flow and oxygenation of their muscles for better endurance while taking advantage of plant food's anti-inflammatory effect to speed their post-workout recovery.** When Tennis star Venus Williams was diagnosed with Sjögren's syndrome, an autoimmune condition, a whole food vegan diet helped her defeat the condition and get back into winning form. Other athletes, such as NFL football stars Tom Brady and Tony Gonzales have been able to extend their careers. At the age of 88, Fred Distelhorst was the oldest man to climb Mt. Kilmanjaro, one of the world's highest peaks and at the ages of 68 and 64, Jannette and Alan Murray circled Australia by running 365 marathons in a year!

CONCLUSIONS:

A Although we do have the choice between omnivore and herbivore, we do our best when we begin to substitute Whole Food Plants for meat.

B Sustainable ideal levels of LDL (BAD) cholesterol is only seen in herbivores.

C Ideal normal average weight is mostly seen among herbivores.

D The healthiest human gut bacteria is found in herbivores.

E The healthiest and longest living people are found in Plant Based societies.

"In our culture, behaving like an omnivore may be normal…but it's also normal to be sick"

BELIEVING SHOULD LEAD TO KNOWING

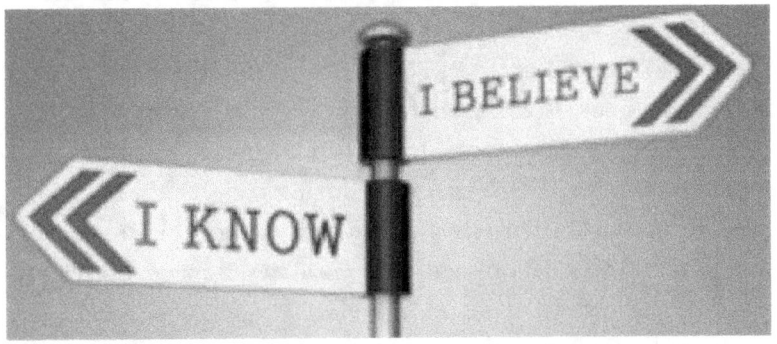

Until that time when you "know" for sure that a certain way of eating is working for you and giving the positive health results you want, you are most probably in the mode of believing. Maybe you're trying a diet out because of a book or article you read or someone you know told you about it or it's the latest "craze." As the old adage says, "people like to hear good news about their bad habits", so they search for a diet plan that resembles what they're presently consuming and therefore requires a minimum of effort to change...regardless of the long term health results. At that point you're trusting blindly because you don't really know for sure if the specific diet will work or not. That's why it's important that believing eventually leads to knowing because, if it doesn't, you might end up hopping from one failed diet to another...endlessly (Wikipedia lists more than 90 different diets). However, once you know, for you the search and experimentation is over. You have found a nutrition path that works for you. Case closed. Now, instead of the need to continue checking out different options, you have a wonderful opportunity to achieve optimal health and wellbeing...based upon a foundation of "knowing"

My suggestion is, before you decide on a particular diet to follow, do the research and find out more about the person who actually created the diet, including, believe it or not, his or her physical appearance. If doctors or nutritionists are promoting diets for the heart or for losing weight, do they look healthy and trim or are they overweight? It may not seem that important but I go along with *practice what you preach*. For example, if a cardiologist is obese or overweight, chances are that he or she will favor medicines over diet. You have to decide what you want.

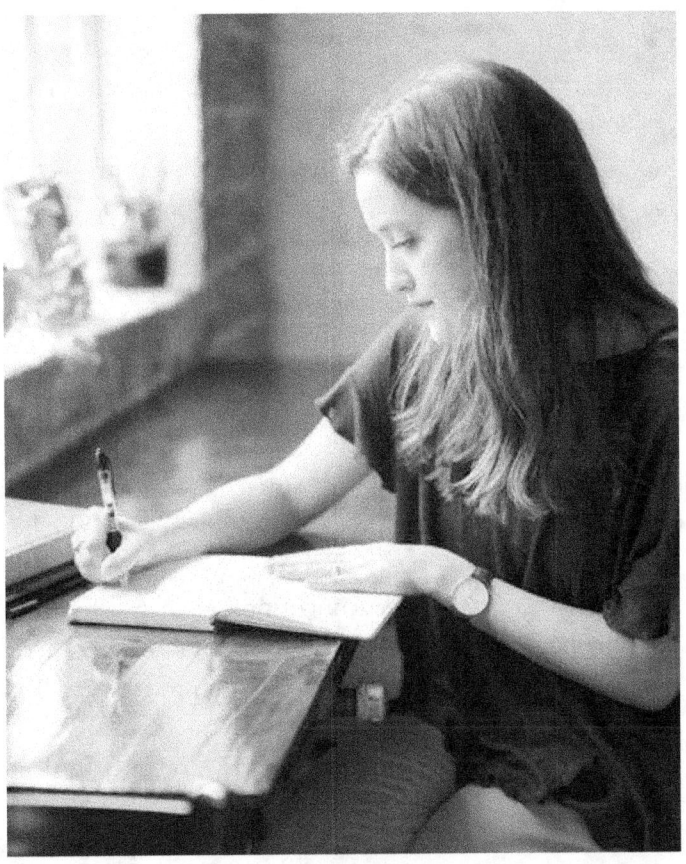

WHEN SELECTING A PARTICULAR DIET IT IS IMPORTANT TO CONSIDER THE FOLLOWING QUESTIONS:

- What facts, studies or investigations are they basing their diet on?
- Who is funding the studies that support the diet?

- What is the history of the diet (i.e., a diet in existence for 5 or 10 years will hardly be able to predict long term health results)?
- What is the author selling (books, vitamins, courses) and do these products indicate a bias towards what they're promoting?

A TIP: Since doing the above investigation can be time consuming and even require certain expertise and training, I'm happy to share with you the following option:

Dr. Michael Greger, the author of the NY Times Best Seller "How Not to Die", is an internationally recognized speaker and expert on nutrition, food safety and public health issues.

His website, http://www.nutritionfacts.org is nonprofit and science based. He provides free daily videos and articles. Every year, his team of volunteers research more than 10,000 nutrition studies. In other words, he does the investigation and research for us. Once on his site you can search any health and nutrition topic.

WHEN DOES A LIE BECOME THE TRUTH?

"A lie told once remains a lie, but a lie told a thousand times becomes the truth."

Do you know who said this?

It is a quote from Joseph Goebbels, who served as Propaganda Minister for Adolph Hitler.

Case in point: "Duck and cover"

For those of us, in our late 60s or 70s, we probably remember that phrase. It was the signal given to us by our teachers, to quickly get under our desks and cover our heads…in order to save us from a nuclear bomb blast. In other words, my flammable wooden desk became my bomb shelter. Today, it sounds so ridiculous and naive that one could only wonder how we actually fell for it…but we did. Not only the students, but I assume that my teacher believed this as well, although I never looked up to see if she ducked under her desk, which happened to be a much bigger bomb shelter than mine. This concept was fed to us by the U.S. Department of Civil Defense, under the guise of protecting us, and we were all gullible enough to go "baa."

Was it a lie?… propaganda?… or just plain ignorance? Who or what was really behind it all?

I'm sure that every reader of this article has an opinion. I personally don't know the answer to that question even though it has given me plenty of food for thought.

Now you may ask, what does all that have to do with the topic of nutrition?

I remember growing up in Brooklyn, N.Y. and eating pretty much whatever my mom put on the table. I never doubted whether or not the food was healthy. I only cared if it was tasty. My father was a butcher so, as you could imagine, we consumed lots of meat and dairy, which was an important part of the basic seven food pyramid that we were taught in school. We learned and believed that 1) meat was the healthiest and most complete source of protein, while plants were not and 2) dairy and especially milk builds strong bones. Maybe we haven't heard these statements a thousand times, but enough times, so that for the great majority of us, they are today accepted as truths and have become part of our culture. Baaaa..

If these two beliefs actually lead to good health and well-being, then that would be wonderful. However, they were so ingrained in us that we have been simply turning a blind eye to all the overwhelming evidence, which shows that the Standard American Diet (SAD) of meat, dairy and processed foods has been leading us down the path of chronic disease and suffering. With almost zero fiber, healthy carbohydrates, antioxidants, phytonutrients and overloaded with saturated fat and cholesterol, following the SAD is detrimental to our health. If we want to get off this unhealthy path we need to start replacing the meat and dairy on our plates with nutrient rich vegetables, fruits and grains.

So how are the two statements about "meat and dairy" related to "duck and cover"? Well, initially we believed both, without questioning whether they were true or not. With regards to the latter, I definitely would not duck under my office desk today if Kim Jong-un decided to launch one. It is perfectly clear to me that "duck and cover" doesn't work. It's just not true. I now have the knowledge and the understanding to make a wise choice, where previously I did not. In the same way, knowing what I now know about "meat and dairy", I now have the power of choice, where previously I did not.

You too now have the power to choose…so choose wisely.

In closing, here is another quite surprising quote from Mr. Goebbels:

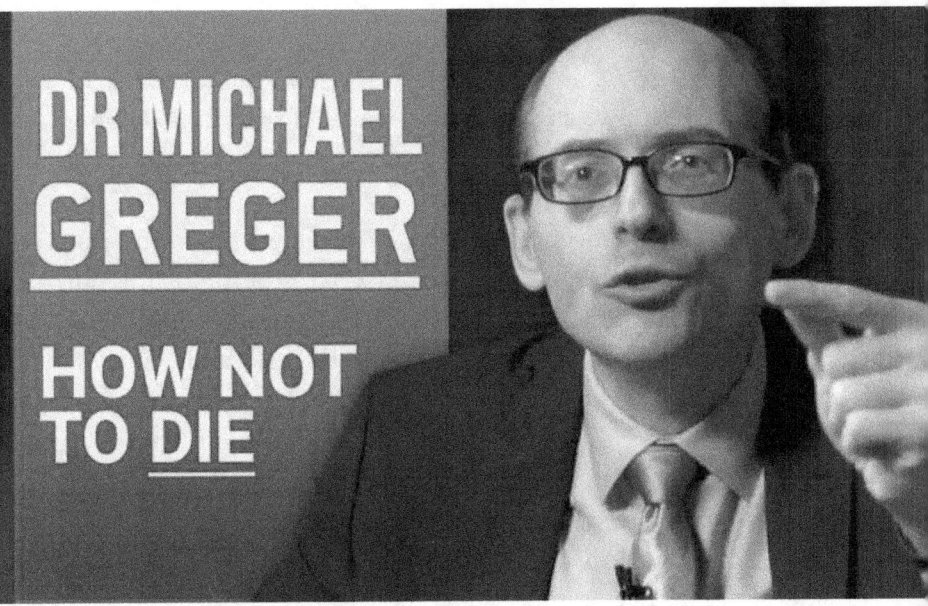

"There will come a day, when all the lies will collapse under their own weight, and truth will again triumph."

INFORMATION IS IMPORTANT BUT FOR THE ESSENTIAL THINGS IN LIFE... WE NEED TO KNOW
PART 1

I saw this sentence on the cover of a book I just read and thought it would be a good way to start this post, especially because of how we are being bombarded by information every moment...information that comes from others, the internet, our cell phones, TV, newspapers, etc. And every moment we need to choose what to believe from this myriad influx of ideas. As a result we carve our way through this life following one or another belief, many times not knowing how they will indeed affect us.

Yet, somewhere along the way we need to transform what we believe into what we know or else we'll be pinballing all over the place, bouncing from one belief to another and this is really important with regards to one of the essential things in life…our physical health.

Previously, I listed 36 different diet options that run from the unknown diets (i.e., Hacker's Diet, Hallelujah Diet, Breatharian Diet, etc.) to the very popular ones (i.e., Atkins Diet, Paleo Diet, Mediterranean Diet, etc.) and if we just consider that number of options it could be quite confusing, especially if your hopping around from one diet to another without getting much satisfaction and unable to reach your goals… long term.

At this time I would like to present to you a known fact:

Populations worldwide that follow a whole food vegan diet (i.e. rural China and Japan and parts of Africa) rarely suffer from the same diseases that are rampant in western societies (heart disease, cancer, diabetes, etc.).

Dr. Michael Greger, on diet and heart disease, from his book "How Not to Die", a NY Times best seller, writes:

"The extraordinarily low rates of heart disease in rural China and Africa have been attributed to the extraordinarily low levels of Cholesterol

among these populations. Though Chinese and African diets are very different, they share commonalities: They are both centered on plant-derived foods, such as grains and vegetables. By eating so much fiber and so little animal fat, there total cholesterol levels averaged under 150mg/dL, similar to people who eat contemporary plant based diets.

An LDL (bad cholesterol) level of 70mg/dL corresponds to a total cholesterol reading of 150, the level below which no deaths from coronary heart disease were reported in the famous Framingham Heart Study, a generations-long project to identify risk factors for heart disease. The population target should therefore be a total cholesterol level under 150mg/dL. "If such a goal was created," Dr. Roberts (author of the Study) wrote, "the great scourge of the western world would be essentially eliminated."

I think that it's about time that we humans take our heads out of the sand and pay attention to the simple fact that people and cultures on the Standard American Diet, with their pharmaceutical drugs, supplements and all the advances in medical technology and research, continue to suffer and die from diseases that almost don't exist among people and cultures on a WFPB diet.

The question is, why is this simple and critical information and all it implies, not common knowledge?

A Is it because the people we rely on and trust don't know this information?

B Is it because they really do know and don't want us to know this information?

C Could it be both A and B?

INFORMATION IS IMPORTANT BUT FOR THE ESSENTIAL THINGS IN LIFE... WE NEED TO KNOW
PART 2

I have a friend who has Parkinson's disease and recently she was upset and depressed that her teeth were starting to become loose. So she went to the doctor that has been treating her illness for the past few years and was told that it's part of the evolution of the disease. He insisted that she begin consuming more dairy products such as milk, cheese and yogurt, because of her body's need for calcium. Since she has been making more effort to eat a whole foods plant based diet, I became concerned over the doctor's insistence since I am completely convinced, from the latest research as well as my own experience, that dairy is quite unhealthy and, contrary to the myth we have been taught since grade school, definitely doesn't "build strong bones and teeth." The truth is, that countries with the highest incidence of osteoporosis (United States, Great Britain, Finland, Australia, etc.) are also the biggest dairy consumers.

According to Dr. John McDougall:

"The incidence of PD is relatively high throughout Europe and North America. In contrast, rural Africans, Chinese, and Japanese, whose diets tend to be vegan or quasi- vegan, have substantially lower rates. The observation that incidence of PD is similar in African-Americans and in whites, all of whom eat the Western diet, further indicates that environmental factors, not race or genetics, are responsible for PD.

Specific foods have been targeted. For example, the consumption of milk in midlife was found to be associated with subsequent development of PD. Men who consume more than two glasses of milk have twice the incidence of PD as men who do not drink cow's milk. The American Cancer Society's Cancer Prevention Study II Nutrition Cohort study has found almost twice the incidence of PD in the highest consumers of milk."

and…

Dr. Michael Greger on how not to die from Parkinson's Disease in his book "How not to die": explains that pollutants such as PCBs, which damage the brain, are still found in higher concentrations in the brains of Parkinson's patients, even though many of these chemicals were banned decades ago. *"You can continue to be exposed to them through the consumption of animal products in your diet, including dairy. Indeed, people who eat dairy free, plant based diets were found to have significantly lower blood levels of the PCBs implicated in the development of Parkinson's disease."*

As a consequence of my friend's doctor prescribing dairy, I decided to do a little bit of research on the internet regarding PD and dental problems and found that, most often, the probable cause of this "side effect" could actually be the medicines themselves and not necessarily the lack of calcium. If the doctor was aware of the potential downside of dairy for Parkinson's patients maybe he could have considered other options such as 1) taking a bone density test for signs of osteoporosis, 2) having the patient see her dentist or 3) even prescribing a calcium supplement. But he didn't. Instead he prescribed dairy.

So, this brings us back to my question in Part 1 of my last post

A) Is it because the people we rely on and trust don't know this information?

The answer seems to be yes! And who do we trust the most? DOCTORS.

And why don't they know? Well, to a great extent it's because of their lack of information regarding the power of nutrition in preventing and reversing diseases. In other words, during those long years preparing to be a doctor, the study of nutrition was almost nonexistent in the great majority of medical schools. . As a result, most medical doctors do not know what their patients should eat to prevent, treat, and often cure chronic diseases, including Parkinson's. So, unless they took it upon themselves to investigate the power of nutrition on their own (post-graduation), how would they know? In other words the doctor is ignorant and the catch phrase "Ignorance is bliss" doesn't really work here…especially for my friend.

And now onto question

B) Is it because they (doctors) really do know and don't want us to know this information?

It's easy to lose sight of the obvious, that the practice of medicine is a business and physicians work for profit. One of the conflicts that many doctor 's face is, while the information becomes more and more conclusive that a healthy diet including lots of fruits, vegetables and grains would be beneficial to the patient, there's the reluctance of suggesting a too "extreme" diet for fear of "turning the patient off" and losing them and $ to another doctor who would let them continue with their bad habits. After 7 years of rigorous schooling it's just bad business. After all, in the end there's always the pills to "cure" what's ailing you…so why bother with offering diet as an option.

IS IT THE AGE?

A friend of mine wanted to know about a physical problem she had regarding a plaque build-up within her aorta artery that

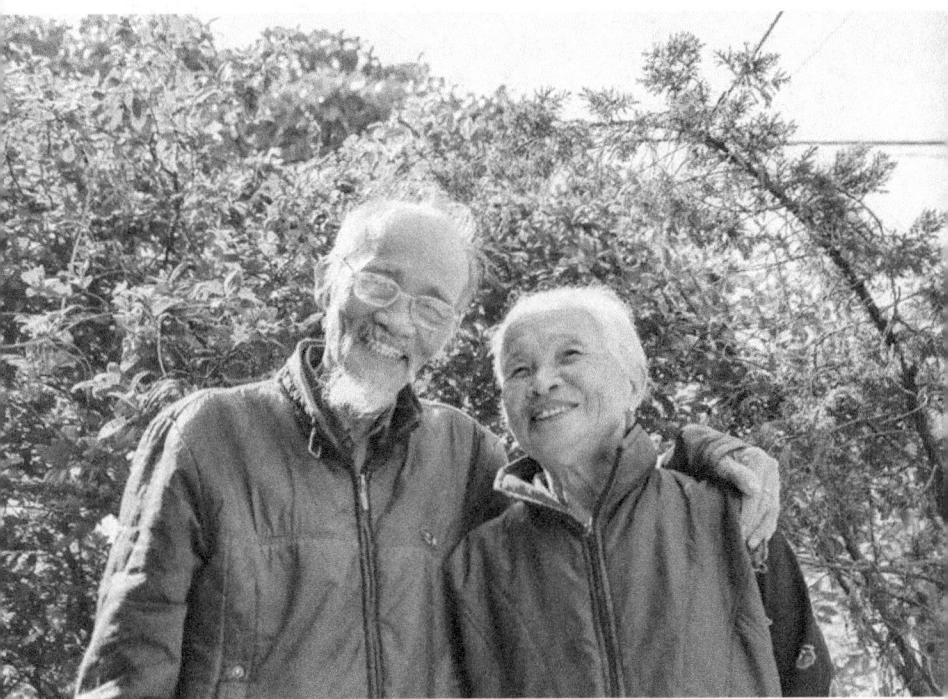

showed up after tests were done. Afterwards, she was told by her cardiologist not to worry about it …that plaque buildup **"is quite normal as you age."** Have you heard that one before? I have. About 10 years ago I took a bone density test and was diagnosed with osteopenia, a pre-cursor to osteoporosis. When I took the results to my physical therapist, who was also an MD, she said that the loss of bone density is a normal consequence of aging. That I shouldn't worry about it. Not only have I heard statements like that from Drs. and caregivers, but friends and family often reply the same way when talking or complaining about some illness they have…**"It's the age."** And it's not only plaque buildup or osteoporosis that is often blamed on age, but high blood pressure, rheumatoid arthritis, dementia and the buildup of cholesterol, as well.

I'm not saying that as we get older we're not more susceptible to the body breaking down, but to write certain diseases off as a **"natural"** result of aging means that there's little we can do about it, so we might as well accept our fate, whatever that illness might be. At the age of 77 I'm well aware of the importance of taking better care of myself because of the wear and tear my body has gone through during my ¾ of a century on the planet. But I'm definitely not going to throw my hands up and accept what fate has to offer. It's like **"climate change."** If you believe it's a natural process of nature and man has nothing to do with it then you will just accept destiny and whatever catastrophes might come along. However, if you see that humans are at least partially responsible for "climate change", then there is hope. Now there is something that can be done…there is action that can be taken to improve the health of our planet. Are we willing to take the risk and do nothing? I don't think that's a good choice.

Similarly, if we don't accept **"It's the age"** adage, doors open for us and now we have options. There are now choices to be made and actions to be taken...if indeed we want to improve our own health. I believe that a long and healthy life is largely a matter of the choices we make.

In 2015, *Dr. Kim Williams* became president of the American College of Cardiology. He was asked why he chose to eat a strictly plant based diet. **"I don't mind dying,"** Dr. Williams said. **"I just don't want it to be my fault."**

THERE ARE TWO TYPES OF PEOPLE... IN THE WORLD OF NUTRITION

To begin, I'd like to share a short story:

Once upon a time there lived two ants, who were close friends. One lived on a salt hill and the other on a sugar hill. One day the ant on the salt hill invited his ant friend, from the

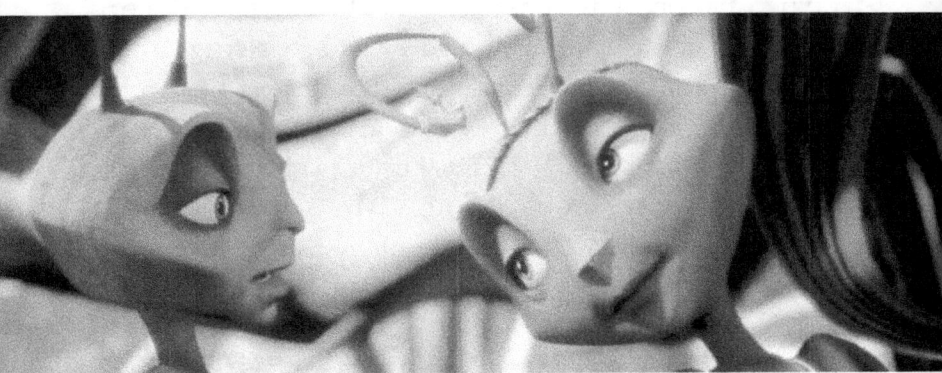

sugar hill, to visit him and to taste his salt. His friend from the sugar hill accepted the invitation and the following day he paid his friend a visit. "Try my salt" he insisted. The sugar ant was not impressed and said, "I would like to invite you to taste my sugar, which is fantastic." So, the next day the salt ant decided to pay him a visit. However, since he had never tasted sugar before, he decided to put a piece of salt in his mouth... just in case he didn't like the sugar. When he arrived, he was offered a grain of sugar and put it in his mouth. "This tastes just like my salt", he said. "That's impossible", the sugar ant replied. He then said, "Open your mouth." He saw the piece of salt and told his guest to remove it. "Now try it." Upon tasting the sugar, the salt ant said, "Yes, your sugar is much tastier than my salt."

The Moral: Sometimes, to learn or accept something new, we need to let go of the old.

So, what are the 2 types of people in the world... of nutrition?
A type 1 person finds it easy to let go of a belief, an idea or a habit, in order to learn something new, or begin a new experience. He or she is usually convinced, from the get go, that the possibilities being offered are well worth the effort involved. At least it's worth giving it a try This was obviously not the case with the ant from the salt hill. Type 2 (the salt ant) has difficulty doing this and, thus, the process of letting go and starting anew, is not easy, because of doubt, fear, etc. With regards to nutrition, changing from the Standard American Diet (SAD) to a Whole Food Plant Based diet (WFPB), would

be easier for type 1. He or she could make the change completely and quickly, whereas type 2 could not. I think that what type we are depends on how we generally react to our life's situations.

I often consider myself Type 1 because, once something makes sense to me and I make a decision to change, there's usually no turning back. Case in point: During the 1970s, while living in Mexico, I was smoking up to 2 packs of cigarettes a day... cigarettes without filters (in Mexico there are a couple of non-filter options). I was also eating lots of meat, dairy and eggs. In 1976 I began exploring the benefits of WFPB nutrition. It was also around that time that the surgeon general published the warning that linked smoking with cancer. So, I decided to quit smoking and, "to kill 2 birds with one stone", on that same day, I also gave up eating meat...and that was it.

Just as I had done, I know people who were able to give up smoking at the snap of the fingers (type 1). I also know people who had to be weaned off of the habit by gradually reducing the quantity, by using smokeless cigarettes, chewing nicotine laced gum or by applying patches (type 2). Whatever type we are, both can be successful...if we decide to switch from the SAD to WFPB nutrition. Why, because I'm convinced that the closer we get to a WFPB diet, the healthier we will be and feel, not only because the research and scientific studies tell us that, but also because of what our taste buds tells us.

THE SECRET IN OUR TASTE BUDS

Unfortunately, it is not common knowledge that once we reach a certain point in our transition from the SAD to a WFPB diet, our taste buds begin to change and remain changed...as we begin to acquire new tastes that are much more compatible with our newly acquired health.

THE SIX BASIC TASTES OF THE HUMAN PALATE:
Sweet ·Salt ·Bitter ·Sour ·Umami ·Fat

Restaurants, especially the fast foods ones, know how to manipulate the combinations of the 3 tastes that we adore most (salt, sweet and fat), into some very enticing foods (i.e., hamburgers, hot dogs, pizza, cheese, ice cream, etc.). Unfortunately, tasty as they are, if we're not careful and aware of the power they can

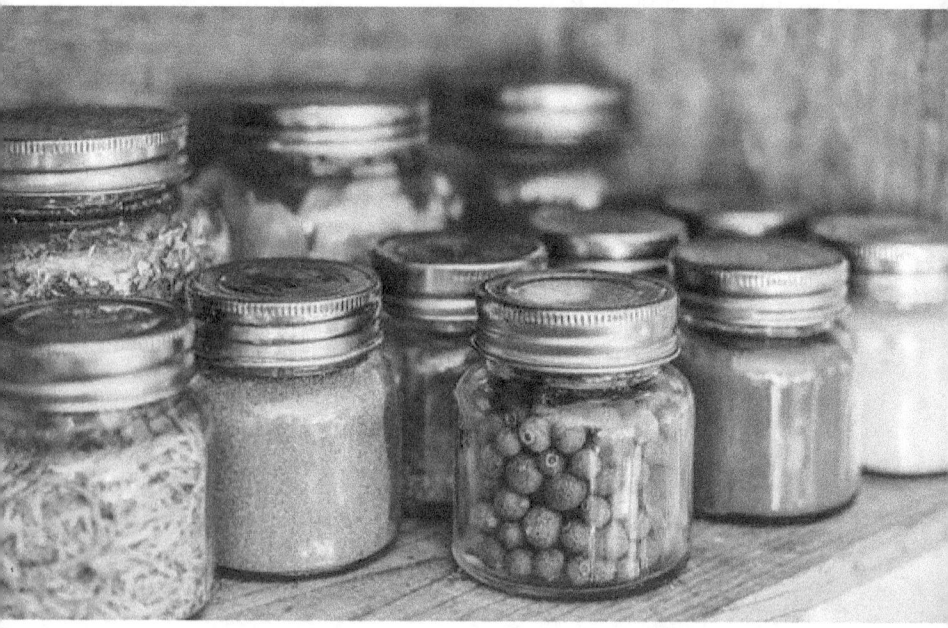

have over us, we can end up strolling unconsciously down a path towards chronic diseases such as heart, cancer and diabetes.

INFORMATION: FRIEND OR FOE?

Born in Brooklyn, New York, I was raised on the *Standard American Diet* with all kinds of meat, dairy, eggs and a great variety of processed and refined foods. My father was a butcher so we had access to all the beef we could ever want and in all forms (i.e., rib steak, tenderloin, spleen, pancreas, bellybutton, ground beef, liver and even cow's brains). We felt very fortunate to have so many "tasty" options at rock bottom prices. Sunday was a very special occasion for the family because of our commitment to a dinner where we literally "overdosed" on pastrami, corn beef, tongue and hotdogs, purchased from the neighborhood Delicatessen. That Sunday evening family meal was so important that all activities were put on hold. My childhood friends knew that, so whether or not we were playing "Hide and Seek" or the military strategic "Ring-a-Levio" or some other group game...once my mother called they would have to go on without me. Of course, at that time during the 1950s, like everyone else, I never thought about the consequences that food could have on my future health. At that time health information was pretty much non-existent. So, just like every kid on the block, I ate what my dear mother put on the table. No questions asked and no doubts came to mind.

Incidentally, during that time, studies were already emerging, linking cigarette smoking with lung cancer. Yet, smoking was widely accepted,

even among doctors, entertainers and sports figures. It would take another 20 years before the public would be informed about cigarettes and cancer. During that time millions of people would die from that disease...which we now know is completely preventable.

The warning labels on cigarette packs are everywhere now, but for a long time, the link between smoking and lung cancer was suppressed by powerful interest groups – much as the relationship between certain foods and other leading killers is suppressed today.

Ever since the 1940s, *The Standard American Diet* (SAD), designed by the Department of Agriculture, has been the foundation of nutrition in Western cultures. Unfortunately,

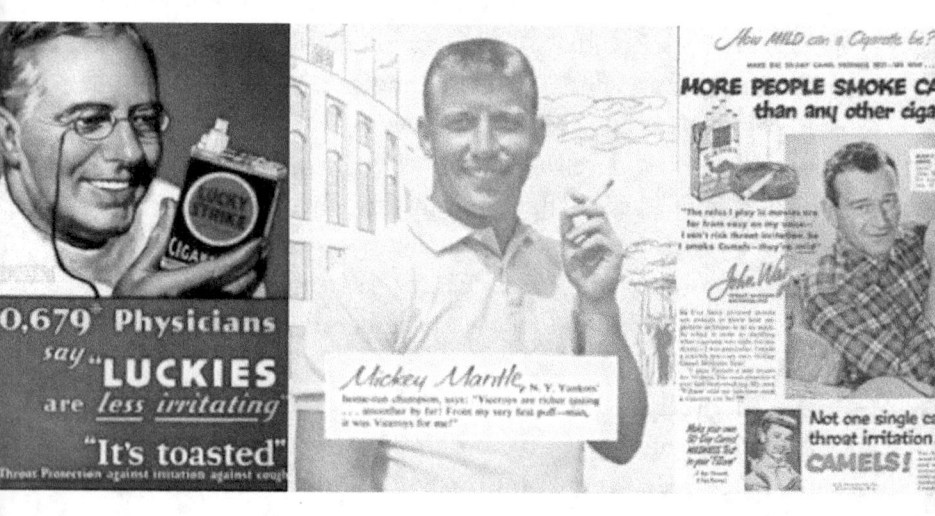

that government organization has always responded to the, not always, health interests of the meat, dairy and eggs industries. As a result, the SAD is what we ate then and still keep eating, to this very day...despite all the contrary health information that's now available in books, videos and on social media. In 1943, the USDA wrote up recommendations called The Basic 7, which included two or more glasses of milk per day for adults and three or four glasses for children. Since then we've had minor changes to that diet, with The Basic Four, The Food Wheel, The Food Guide Pyramid, My Pyramid, and My Plate. Each of these stress a high protein, high fat and low carb diet. The results are a dismal health picture among populations following this diet. We're not only talking about the prevalence of chronic diseases such as heart, cancer, type 2 diabetes, and osteoporosis but illnesses and afflictions such as obesity, high blood pressure, chronic constipation, allergies and auto-immune diseases (i.e., rheumatoid arthritis, multiple sclerosis, type 1 diabetes, inflammatory bowel disease). Mind you...these diseases and afflictions are rare in populations that follow a Whole Food Plant Based (WFPB) diet.

With regards to nutrition, between the 1940s and 1960s the following significant events took place that would forever change the nutrition and health horizon in countries that were dependent on the Standard American Diet:

FACTORY FARMS: With the growth of large cities and people's cravings for meat, dairy and eggs, small farms could no longer keep up with the demand. Thus, the need for a more efficient means of production. The demand for vast quantities of meat at cheap prices led to meat producers pushing for efficiency and squeezing every bit of profit   from every animal. Recently, scores of documentaries and videos have been produced showing the horrific environment and treatment in the factories...where the animals live and die.

HORMONES: In order to fatten the animals, during the 1950s, the Food and Drug Administration (FDA) approved a number of steroid hormone drugs for use in beef cattle and sheep, including natural estrogen, progesterone, testosterone, and their synthetic versions. Studies show that, when consumed, the added hormones can cause serious unbalances within the human body.

ANTIBIOTICS: Because of the need to keep cramped animals in tight and unsanitary conditions, antibiotics in feed have been used in animal production in Europe since 1953 and in the USA since the 1960s. In the 1970s, researchers began warning that routine use of antibiotics was contributing to a surge in drug-resistant germs, or superbugs, that render antibiotics powerless against deadly infections in humans. A study in 1976 showed that highly-resistant e. coli E. coli bacteria could pass from chickens to farm workers who worked with the animals, in just a few weeks.

PESTICIDES: The pesticides used on crops meant for animals on Factory Farms end up embedded in the animal's fat and milk. Those harmful chemicals eventually end up in the food we eat.

So, is the information we get on health and nutrition, friend or foe...a blessing or a curse?

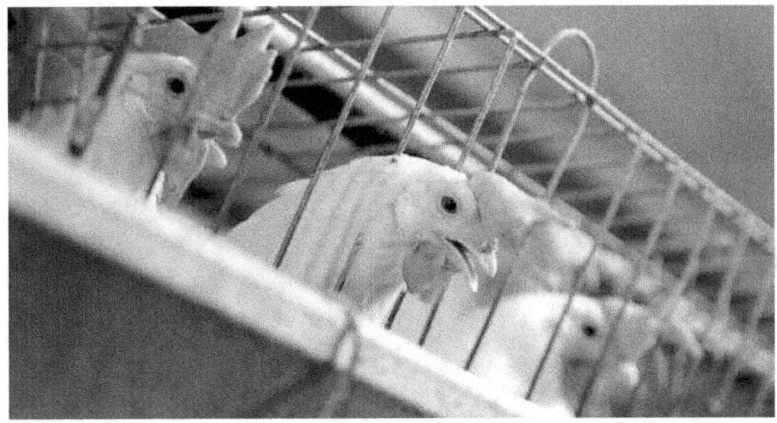

Well, I think that it depends on the source of the information...and that responsibility falls upon each one of us. It's quite obvious that there have always been interest groups trying to control the information we get. Now it's time to wake up to that fact. It's only then that we can begin to decipher who is actually looking out for us. I know that for many people it's not easy to change diet and lifestyle, but once you start reaping the benefits of the changes and notice a difference in your health and wellbeing, the motivation to continue becomes energizing.

IS GOOD HEALTH A WANT OR A NEED?

Recently, I asked this question to several people and they all agreed that Good Health is definitely a need. When I posed a follow-up question: What's the difference between a want and a need? I found that there were differences of opinions.

To distinguish the difference between a want and a need I decided to investigate and came up with the following:

- **A need** is something that is extremely necessary for a person to survive. If a need is not met, it would lead to suffering, the onset of disease, the inability to function effectively and efficiently in society, and even death. Also, needs are the same for everyone.
- **Wants** are desires that are optional, meaning that you will be fine and can still go on living, even if the want is not met. Wants are not the same for everyone and often change over time.

As I found out, we often confuse the two, saying that we "need" something when what we really mean to say is "want" (i.e., I need a new car vs. I want a new car or I need to make more money vs. I want to make more money). As a result, in our daily lives we get used to interchanging these words without giving it a second thought.

There are certain needs that are very obvious, clear and vital to us, and without them death is imminent. These needs follow the law of 3:

1. Air – Death after approximately 3 minutes
2. Water – Death after approximately 3 days
3. Food – Death after approximately 3 weeks

So, is "Good Health" a Want or a Need?
Although it may not be so obvious as the "Big 3", according to the definition above it is a need, because if we're deprived of

Good Health, "it would lead to suffering, the onset of disease, the inability to function effectively and efficiently in society, and even death."

A QUESTION OF TASTES

We all "want" the food we eat to taste good and that's wonderful because that's what our taste buds are made for...to satisfy this "want." However, "tasting good" is in fact very short lived. It ends once we take that last swallow. The flavor of the food we eat lasts only a few minutes...while we're chewing. The food is then passed on to the rest of our body, which responds to the "need" to be nourished. There are no taste buds from the throat down and therefore no taste experience beyond our mouth. Unfortunately, we can get stuck so much on the flavors of the food that we completely forget that for the next few hours our bodies and our immune system will be working incessantly trying to keep us healthy. One example of this is the craving that millions of people around the world have for fast foods, even though they know how unhealthy they are. The want for flavors overshadows the need to be healthy. This craving for taste is so dominant that many people, even those who switch to a plant based diet for health reasons, find it very difficult to give up the cravings for hamburgers, cheeses, pizzas, KFC, etc. They constantly try to find substitutes for those tastes, substitutes that are often highly processed, requiring additives, salt, sugars, trans-fats and artificial coloring, just to mimic the tastes that they are missing. These highly processed substitutes are often not much healthier than the original unhealthy food that people are trying to give up.

In my experience, losing the cravings for different foods takes a while, similar to giving up smoking. Because our taste buds are constantly being renewed, they will eventually adapt and even thrive with the new tastes. We just have to be patient. For example, if we completely refrain from eating salt for one week and then eat something salty, it will taste "too" salty. My suggestion is to not focus on the foods we think we're missing but to focus on the new world of flavors that are awaiting us.

In conclusion, once "Good Health" becomes the priority for us and is recognized as a "need" we will become more aware of the positive or negative repercussions of what we put into our mouths. We will realize that taste, although important and satisfying, is only a small part of the digestive process and that we need to be more diligent and more pro-active by choosing the foods that respond to our body's needs. By the way. By consuming more Whole Food Plant Based foods combined with exercise and stress management we will not only lose weight but also reap in the benefits of excellent health. In other words, "we can have our cake and eat it too."

IN THE END THINGS SHOULD MAKE SENSE TO US

"There are lies, there are damn lies and there are statistics"

Mark Twain (1845 – 1910)

This quote from one of America's favorite authors really caught my eye and as I read it over and over again, something popped

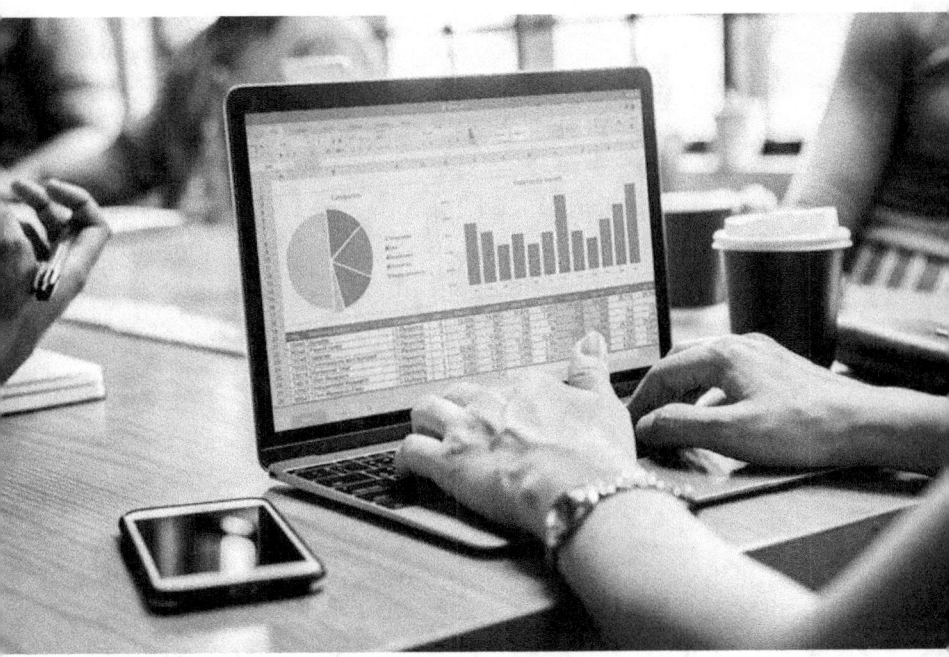

out. Here is this man from the 19th century stating that statistics can be bigger lies than just lies and damn lies. I asked myself "How bad could statistics have been in the 19th century? I mean, weren't people more simple and therefore, more honest back then? Then I thought: "Imagine if Mr. Twain was alive today." What would he say about today's statistics?" Today's world is run on statistics…from politics to economics to the social media to health and nutrition. Where doesn't statistics have it's finger in the pie?

CAN WE DEPEND ON STATISTICS?

If we go back to Mark Twain's time, during the 1800s, we find that one use of statistics was to show the unemployment rate in the U.S. These statistics however were based only on people who were actively looking for work. It did not include people who stopped looking or, in fact, were not working at all. In other words, it did not reflect the total unemployment rate of the country, which would have been higher. Why was it done? Well, because it functioned well politically. Interestingly, that same system of determining the unemployment rate, is still being utilized today...150 years later. Manipulation?

STATISTICS AND NUTRITION

So how do those tactics relate to what's happening today in the world of nutrition? Well, there are multi-billion dollar industries that have so much invested in their products that they can't afford to lose clients and profits. Their stockholders won't tolerate that. Just as the tobacco companies manipulated statistics, during the mid-20th century, to battle the thousands of studies showing the link between smoking and cancer, today there are numerous corporations and industries doing similar things. If their bottom line is being threatened, they can finagle the statistics in order to convince their customers that things are humming along just fine. Because the stakes are so high, the ends are often justified by the means. For me, just as important as it is to read the ingredients listed on the foods we buy, for health reasons, we should also question who the authors or sponsors are behind nutrition research and studies. Why? Because of the problem of bias.

IN THE END THINGS SHOULD MAKE SENSE TO US

Since Whole Food Plant Based nutrition is my passion and I have a genuine desire to help people improve their health,

I am concerned about how statistics are confusing us? With so much conflicting information, from health care professionals, our family, friends and especially the social media, how can we be sure if the information is valid. This is especially important when we need to make important decisions regarding our health. Yes, statistics are important but what's equally important, in my opinion, is that our decisions are based upon what "makes sense" to us. When it does, a decision that may have appeared complicated and doubtful at first, all of a sudden, becomes simple and clear. For, when something makes sense to us there's an understanding that touches us in such a way that we can say with conviction...yes "That Makes Sense!"

EATING HEALTHY IS SIMPLE, IT'S JUST NOT ALWAYS EASY

I have been watching my cat a lot more these days and one thing I notice about his eating habits is that he knows what he likes and seems to like what's good for him. For Gin (that's his name), eating is a simple matter since he eats pretty much the same thing every day. I assume that it's that way for cats and dogs everywhere. I remember going to the zoo when I was younger, and saw that lions, tigers and bears, as well as elephants, crocodiles, and seals ate the same thing every day. Although I've never been on an African safari I do get the opportunity of watching wildlife documentaries and I see that, in the wild, animals know exactly what to eat and will stick to their regimen, no matter what. There is no confusion. Nature has conveniently programmed animals to specific diets.

What happens when an animal goes off it's natural diet?
Examples of this can be found with animals that are raised on factory farms (i.e., cows, pigs and fish) where their diets are compromised.

> *"A Cows Natural Diet consists of plants that can be "grazed" or "browsed." Grazing generally refers to the eating of grasses, and browsing usually refers to the eating of leaves, twigs, or bark from bushes or trees. Cows both graze and browse, but they are definitely more "grazers" than "browsers" and their complicated four-part stomach helps them to slowly digest relatively large amounts of grasses. From a historical perspective, consumption of ground grains has NOT been part of the cows' natural diet."*

This is what you might find on small farms where cows are grass-fed. When factory farms sprung up during mid-19th century, because of the growing consumer demand for meat, grass fed cows were no longer feasible. There just wasn't enough grazing land available and so it wasn't profitable. The diet had to change and large amount of grains such as corn and soy substituted the grass. It also helped to fatten the cows which resulted in a greater profit margin. Also, a grass fed cow has less fat and more muscle than a grain fed cow and as a result…the meat is usually tougher.

Unfortunately, this unnatural diet combined with the claustrophobic conditions of the factory farms has led to diseases and infections among the cows. That resulted in the use of antibiotics as an attempt to control the diseases, although not always with success. Factory farm pigs and fish are also not eating the foods that nature intended them to eat.

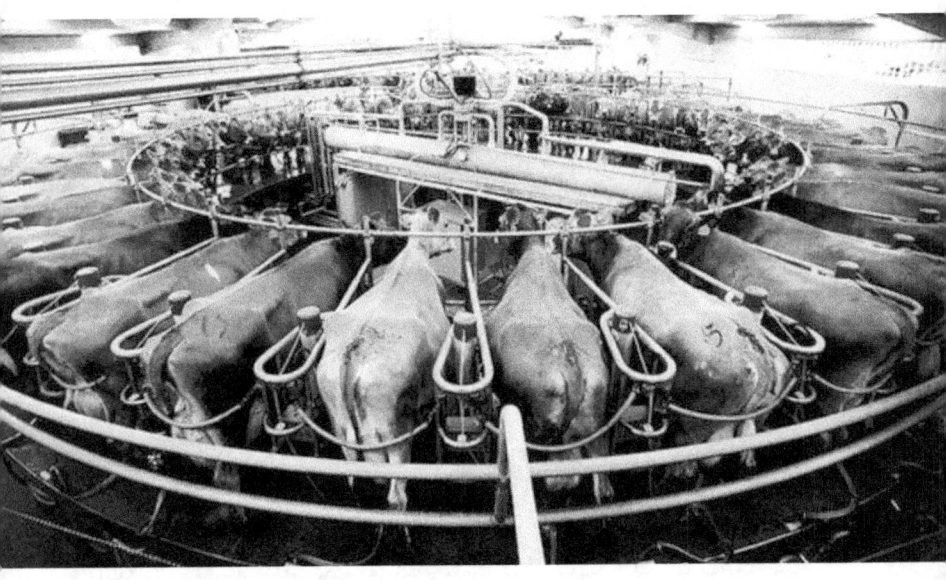

So what has this to do with humans?

Since animals know what their natural food is…why isn't that the case with humans? Why are there so many contradictions and why has it become so complicated that Wikipedia lists 93 different diets. Isn't it possible that, as with the diseases on factory farms, one of the main reasons for chronic diseases among us humans is simply because we're not eating what nature meant us to eat?

WHAT DOES HISTORY TELL US?

1) Populations that mostly eat plant based foods (i.e., rural China, Japan, and parts of Africa – Nepal and Kenya – where long distant champion runners come from) rarely suffer from the chronic diseases that

plague people on the Standard American Diet (SAD) of meat, dairy and processed foods. These populations have been eating plant based for centuries. Also, they don't use supplements, count calories, worry about sugar or salt intake or have problems with gluten or carbohydrates. They eat what their ancestors ate. For them, eating healthy is simple and easy.

2) According to Dan Buettner's book "The Blue Zones", the longest living people on the planet eat plant based foods (i.e., Okinawa, Japan, Sardinia, Italy, Loma Linda, California, Ikaria, Greece and the Nicoya Peninsula, Costa Rica).

3) The Tarahumara Indians in Northern Mexico are considered "the modern Spartans," because of their amazing endurance. They can run races day and night, kicking a ball for 100 miles, for the fun of it. According to the research: "Probably not since the days of the ancient Spartans (of Greece) has a people achieved such a high state of [extreme] physical conditioning." And what do they eat? A diet made up of 75 to 80 percent starch (carbohydrates) based on "beans, corn, and squash."

4) When healthy people from regions that consume plant based foods change their diets when they move to regions that consume the Standard American Diet, they begin to suffer the SAD diseases (i.e., heart, cancer, diabetes, osteoporosis, high blood pressure, obesity).

5) *Recently, the remains of dozens of Roman gladiators were discovered in a mass grave. Using just their skeletons, they were able to reconstruct the death blows, show just how strong they really were, and even reconstruct their "diet of barley and beans." They were actually called "hordearii" which meant "Barley Men." Similarly, the Roman army troopers, famed for their fighting abilities, also were eating a similar kind of diet, suggesting "The best fighters in the ancient world were essentially vegetarian."*

It's important to recognize that fad diets have only been in existence for decades…at most! and so they can only make health claims based on short term results. Compare that to the successful track record of civilizations consuming plant based foods, that have been around for thousands of years.

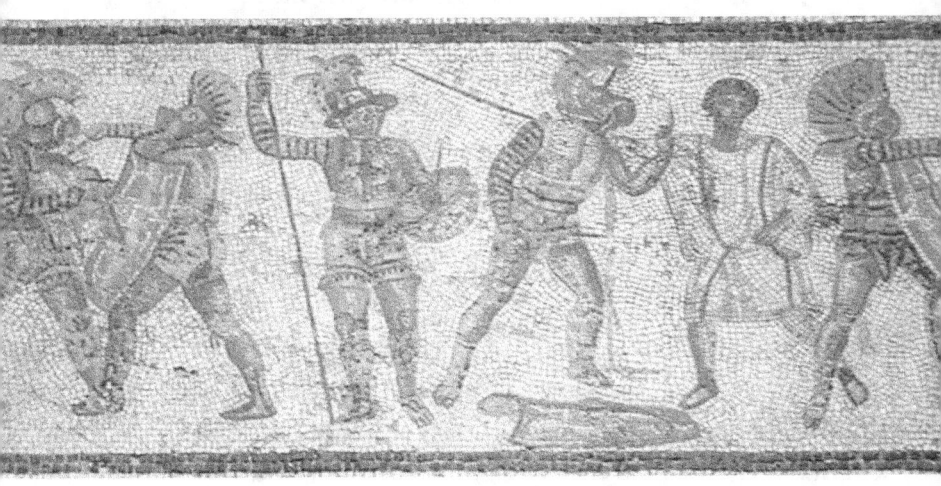

SO WHY ISN'T EATING HEALTHY EASY?

Because we live in a consumer society we are faced with a constant barrage of enticing products that we are expected to buy into. Marketing experts are trained to capture our attention with the latest and greatest products and fads. This is especially true in the field of nutrition because there's nothing closer to us then what we put in our mouths. Unfortunately, most marketing experts are motivated primarily by sales and to a lesser extent...our health. As a result of their persistent efforts to sell us their products, we end up in a never ending cycle of confusion about what foods are healthy for us. As a result, the choices that we make regarding nutrition may not be in our best interest. Understanding the essence of nature, it seems to make sense to me that human beings had always known perfectly well how to feed itself, just as all other species know how to feed themselves. Yet, because this nutrition "knowledge" has been forgotten, we end up believing so called diet "experts" who happen to have written a book or two on nutrition. As long as we're in the mode of believing...we will never know. We need to connect again with the knowledge that lies within us...that would reveal what foods are best for us.

OUR BODY IS WHERE THE GIFT OF LIFE RESIDES

I have always felt that our greatest gift is the gift of life. Yes, we have the gifts of sight and hearing, the ability to think and imagine and to feel joy and love, among other things. But, none of this would be possible if we hadn't first received the gift of life. However, I'd like to call your attention to another

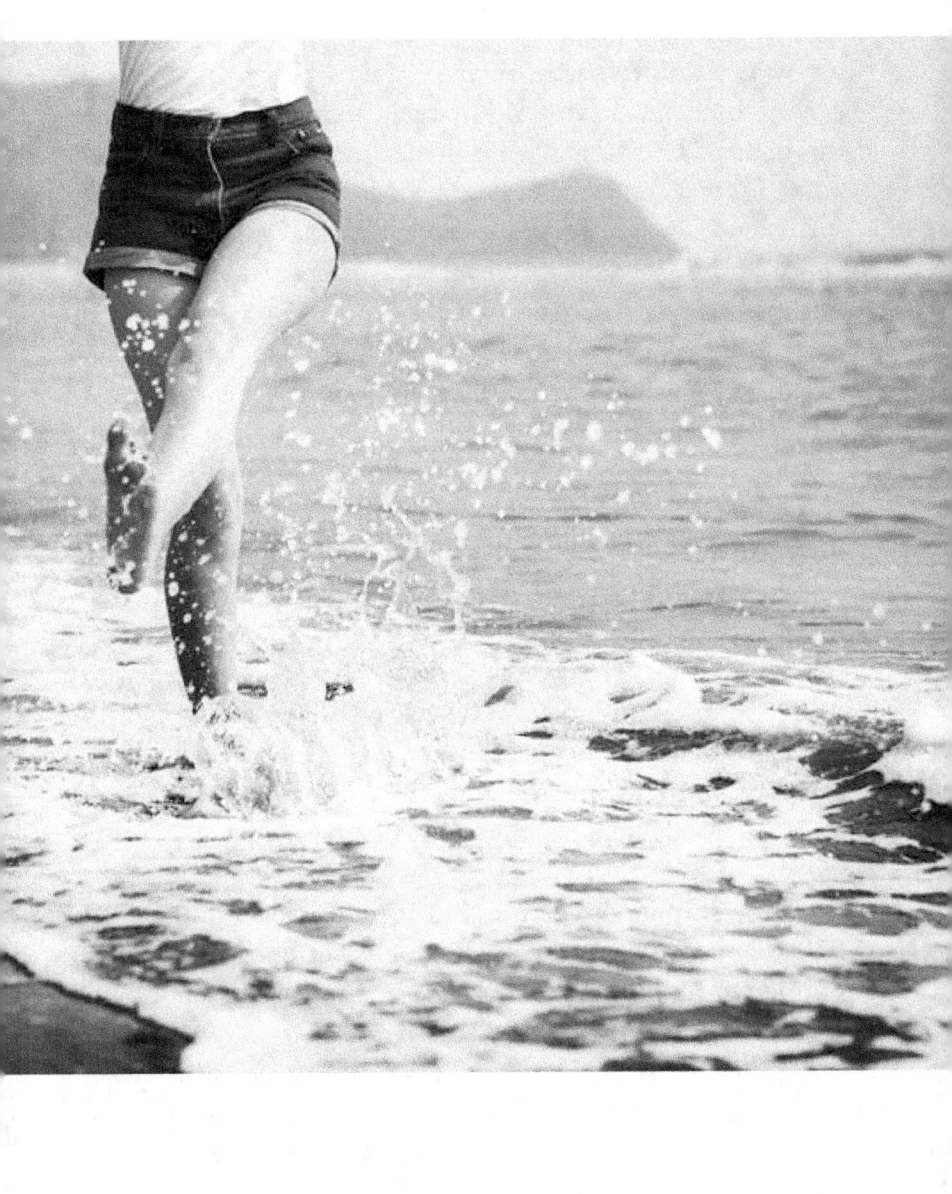

gift, which unfortunately we don't often see as a gift, and that is this container or vessel or temple... called the body. It is through the body that we experience the gift of life. Without it, life for you and me could not happen.

A few days ago, a friend of mine had a severe heart attack, which fortunately she survived. She contacted me because of my personal experience with a Whole Food Plant Based (vegan) diet which, for the past 8 years, I have highly recommended to anyone interested in achieving optimal health. I offered to lend her an extraordinary book by Dr. Caldwell Esselstyn, the NY Times Best Seller, "Prevent and Reverse Heart Disease." In the end however she commented that her situation was not that bad and that going vegan would be too extreme at this time. Anyway, that got me thinking. Changing to a Whole Food Plant Based diet for many people is considered extreme. The word "Vegan" is often associated with fanaticism and "Veganism" is considered by some as akin to a "religion" which they don't want to be converted to. That would mean having to give up their favorite foods, whether or not those foods were healthy in the first place.

Anytime someone tells me that Whole Food Plant Based (WFPB) nutrition is too extreme I experience an "inner" giggle...for 2 reasons:

1) *What would actually be extreme to me is laying on an operating table and having a surgeon saw through my ribs and stopping my heart in order to replace a clogged artery or two. That's extreme!*

2) *Eating tasty and easy to prepare plant based foods is so simple these days. There are thousands of recipes available now on the internet and in books that can easily replace some of the unhealthy foods that we're accustomed to.*

DON'T BE TURNED OFF BY "DARK THOUGHTS"

Have you ever had the desire of doing something or accomplishing a task or a job that was a challenge but you wanted to do it anyway...against all odds? Then someone close to you commented, for whatever reason, that what you want to do would be impossible or risky and that you shouldn't even try it; so you decided not to. You just gave up. During a conference I attended several years ago the guest speaker used the term "Dark Thoughts" to describe that very situation. It's when someone says that something cannot be done, even though it's never been tried before, especially by him or her. How does that relate to WFPB nutrition? Well, you may have the desire or need to eat healthier but "dark thoughts" from your own mind, or from someone else's, may try to convince you not to do it...even though you know that it would be the correct decision. It takes courage to say NO to dark thoughts!

IT'S NOT "ALL OR NOTHING AT ALL"

One thing I've learned during these past 8 years on a WFPB diet is that some people are able to make the switch easily and never turn back while, for others, the change needs to be gradual. I'm not sure if it's will power or simply a difference in personalities. I became attracted to vegetarianism in 1976, basically because of my interest in oriental philosophy and not so much for health reasons. So, one day I decided to give up meat and that was it. And, to "kill two birds with one stone", that same day I gave up smoking. For me it wasn't difficult. That's the way I am. However, for a lot of people, giving up smoking and animal products, such as meat and dairy, takes time…and that's OK too.

So when I say: It's Not, "All or Nothing at All" it means that there are two choices:

1) *Make the switch once and for all to a WFPB diet in order to best prevent chronic diseases in the future or,*

2) *Take one step at a time, with the same goal of adapting to a WFPB diet, according to your own health needs. For example, a person who is actually suffering from a chronic disease (i.e., heart, cancer, diabetes 2, osteoporosis, high blood pressure), would require a stricter WFPB diet than a person who is not.*

For me, the advantage of making the change once and for all, was to reap the benefits of WFPB nutrition as soon as possible (within a few weeks). The result was an influx of inspiration that helped me to continue along the path. But, that's my situation. If the change is gradual, the benefits will probably be felt gradually. Everyone is different and each person will have to find their own path on the journey to better health. What's important is to take the first step. However, for anyone suffering from a chronic disease, I suggest making the change ASAP.

GLOBAL FOOD IMPERIALISM

Many people around the world are lactose intolerant because they lack the enzyme lactase, which is necessary to digest the sugar in milk and dairy products (lactose). This is especially true in populations that historically rarely consume dairy, such as countries in Asia (i.e., China, Japan, Korea). In Mexico, approximately 50% of the population is lactose intolerant...

History

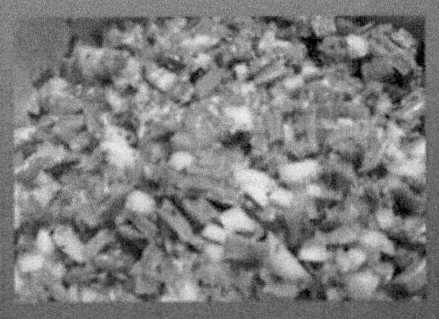

- Spanish Conquistadores arrived in Mexico City

- Diet consists of corn-based dishes with chiles and herbs.

- Beans, nopales and tomatoes

- Indigenous people ate avocados, papaya, guava, jicama

1.
www.gourmetsleuth.com/...Beverages...
/chocolate-mayordomo.aspx

and a large percentage are not aware of it. As a result, many Mexicans, who are lactose intolerant, end up having digestive problems such as stomach and intestinal pain, diarrhea, bloating, nausea and excess gas. They end up taking over the counter and prescription medicines that sometimes alleviate the symptoms…without treating the cause.

So, I began wondering why is it that so many Mexicans, including my wife, are lactose intolerant? Why do so many lack the enzyme to properly digest dairy?

THE FIRST GLOBAL FOOD IMPERIALISTS INVADE MEXICO
– *The Spanish "Conquistadores"*

While the study of the conquest of Mexico and Latin America has generally focused on the social, political, and economic changes forced upon Indigenous populations, the matter of food—the very source of survival—is rarely considered. Yet, food was a principal tool of colonization. Arguably, one cannot properly understand colonization without taking into account the issue of food and eating. When Columbus landed in the Americas, he found that, except for dogs, there were almost no tamed animals…no cattle, goats, horses or sheep. The natives did not raise animals for meat or dairy consumption. What small quantity of meat they did eat was from animals in the wild. Nor did indigenous populations consume milk or any dairy products. This was not only true for Mexico but for almost all native Indians throughout the Americas. Without animals like cows, sheep and goats, the Mexica (Aztec) diet was mainly vegetables, fruit and grains. At the top of the list was corn, an ancient and sacred crop that could grow almost anywhere. The early cultivation of corn, thousands of years ago, allowed all great Meso-American civilizations to flourish. However, since the invading Spanish soldiers were accustomed to meat and dairy, which they consumed back home, they considered the indigenous diet inferior and not very appetizing. So, on his second voyage to the "New World", in 1493, Columbus brought the hoofed animals whose meat would immediately replace the foods that were unacceptable.

What ensued was extraordinary and would fundamentally change the lives of the indigenous people forever. Since the cows, pigs, goats and sheep were new to this world, they had no predators. These imported animals were allowed to roam and graze freely with no threats to their existence. As a result, they reproduced at an astonishing rate. Little by little, the arable land used by the natives was overtaken by the animals and less land was available for the growing of corn, grains, vegetables and fruits. Just as the Spanish settlers found the indigenous food unacceptable, the natives were unable to adapt to the Spanish diet of meat and dairy. Initially, many Indigenous people became malnourished, which consequently weakened their resistance to European diseases. Others literally starved to death as their agricultural plots were trampled, consumed by the animals or appropriated for Spanish crops. In time, many Indigenous people, left with limited options, began to consume European foods in place of the foods that had nourished them for centuries. Just as in Asian countries, where dairy was historically never a part of their diet, the Indians of Mesoamerica also lacked the lactase enzyme. However, as time went by, the Europeans, who were not lactose intolerant, mated with the natives and their offspring, the present day Mexican, has approximately a 50/50 chance of being lactose intolerant.

THE SECOND GLOBAL FOOD IMPERIALISTS ARRIVE IN MEXICO – *NAFTA and the Standard American Diet*

After doing extensive research in order to find out when and how diets changed for the worse in Mexico... changes that

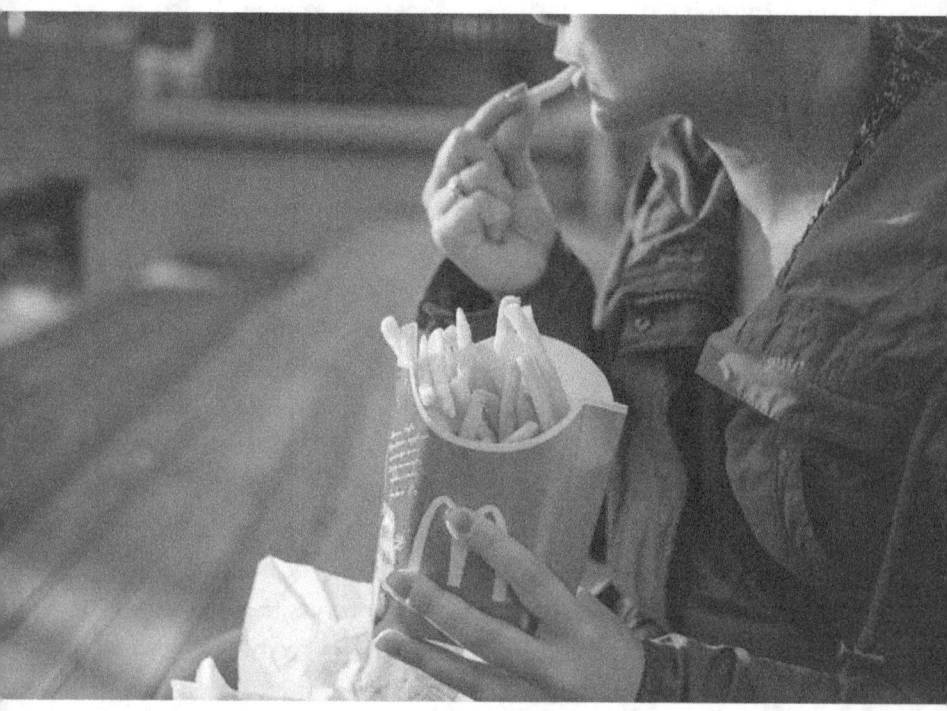

led to tremendous spikes in heart disease, cancer obesity and especially type 2 diabetes, we can return to the end of the 1970s, with the first established Fast Food company from the north...Burger King, in Mexico City. This was followed by McDonalds in 1985. According to an article in the New York Times: *"More than a week after the first McDonald's restaurant opened in Mexico, long lines spilled into the street as people patiently awaited the taste of their first Mexican-made Big Mac. Cars waiting to enter the packed McDonald's parking lot or pass through the novel drive-through window caused mammoth traffic jams along the Periférico Sur, the most important thoroughfare in southern Mexico City."*

However, the "big blow" to Mexico's nutrition, happened as a result of the North American Free Trade Agreement (NAFTA). Trade opened up between the 3 countries (The United States, Canada and Mexico) and although some Mexican farmers profited from exporting certain fruits and vegetables (peppers, tomatoes, mangoes, limes, and avocados), because the production of corn was subsidized by the U.S. government, Mexican farmers couldn't compete with the ridiculously low prices. Eventually more than 2,000,000 corn farmers would be displaced and forced to look for work in large cities and to our northern neighbor. At the same time, corporations in the U.S. that produced highly processed foods, such as...

- **Dairy, from saturated fats**
- **Treats made from refined sugars, salt, oils and conservatives**
- **Processed meats**
- **Sugary drinks**

- **Fried foods**
- **Refined grains**

were now salivating at the opportunity of selling their products to their Southern neighbor. Gradually, these products began to infiltrate the markets and replace the healthier grains, fruits and vegetables that had been the foundation of Mexican cuisine for centuries. This was especially true with regards to packaged junk foods aimed at children.

According to Alyshia Gálvez, a professor of Latin American, Latino, and Puerto Rican Studies at the City University of New York, in her book published this year (2018) by UC Press, EATING NAFTA: Trade, Food Policies, and the Destruction of Mexico, *"Today, Mexico is the largest consumer of carbonated drinks in the world, and the largest consumer of processed foods in Latin America. As has been well-documented, this is one of many causes of a snowballing health crisis. In nearly every country experiencing this sort of economic transition, chronic illnesses including heart disease and diabetes have surpassed communicable diseases."* She goes on to say, *"Basically, both countries (United States and Mexico) are experiencing public health crises, but Mexico's is comparably worse because it exports so much of its produce to the U.S. market. Instead of the tianguis markets where local fruits and vegetables were historically inexpensive and plentiful, the food needs of Mexicans are increasingly met by chains like Walmart, Coca Cola-owned OXXO, and Circle K."*

Although these changes have happened over centuries, because of Food Imperialism, the people of Mexico are now suffering from the chronic diseases that were not so rampant just a few decades ago.

SO, WHAT'S THE FUTURE?

The United States, Canada and Mexico are expecting to sign a trade agreement that will replace NAFTA and hopefully this time there will be more control over the corporations that are currently pushing junk foods into Mexico. A positive trade deal, combined with educating the public on whole food nutrition that is based on the foods our ancestors ate (grains, fruits and vegetables), could mean the beginning of a reversal of the incidence of chronic diseases that cause so much suffering as well as premature death. Historically, in trade agreements, it's usually the technologically advanced nations that get the best of the deal. The challenge is to make sure that this doesn't happen again and that the next trade agreement is a *"win, win"* situation for the people in each country.

HEALTH OR WEALTH...WHAT'S MORE IMPORTANT TO YOU?

For some of you older folks (including me), you might remember the comedian Jack Benny who was very popular on

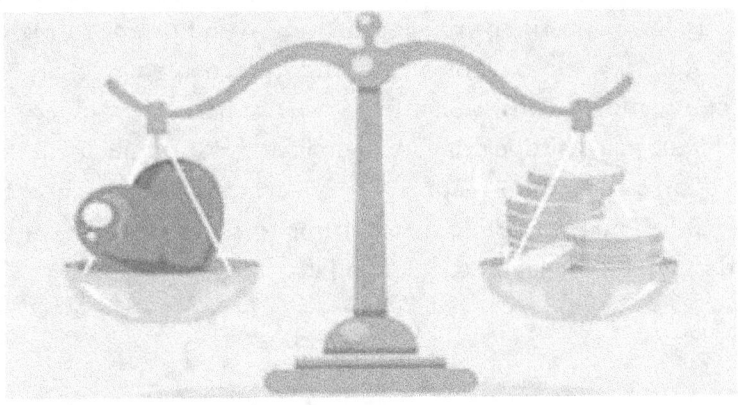

radio and television during the 40s and 50s. Jack was a tight-wad, famous for his extreme stinginess. He tells a story, in one of his skits, that he was walking down an alley and was approached by a robber. Pointing a gun at his head the robber blurted, "Your money or your life!" Jack stood there, stone faced, and silent. Once again, "your money or your life." Again no response. "This is your last chance, your money or your life." Jack, expressionless, stared at the robber and yelled "I'm thinking…I'm thinking!" This joke got a big laugh from the audience. Why? Well because it was obvious that life is more important than money and there's really nothing to think about. It's a "no brainer."

Faced with that same situation, unless you have a black belt in martial arts, I assume that, like me, you would fork over all the money you had. Although health is, obviously, not as vital as the threat of, instantaneously, losing one's life, "can you really enjoy your wealth if you're suffering from a severe illness or a chronic disease?" If your response is no, and I assume it is, then my follow-up question is: "How much time and effort are you actually investing in your health"? As far as I'm concerned, when something is important to me, I invest in it. We know how much time and energy we spend on accumulating wealth…during most of our lives. How much do we dedicate to our health? For so many of us, not much…until of course something happens (i.e., severe illness or chronic disease). Then we decide that it's time to focus on our health, although, by then, it could be too late.

BESIDES WEALTH, DURING OUR LIFETIME WE ALSO INVEST MANY YEARS ON OUR EDUCATION AND OUR CAREERS!

If we wait until later on in life to think about our health, because we're feeling OK, while we're young, one day we may find ourselves in a precarious health situation where we end up saying to ourselves "I should have taken better care of myself."

The solution, in my opinion, is not to wait until the last moment before we focus on our health. What better time to start than right now? And how to start? Begin by increasing the amount of Whole Plant Based Foods in your diet and consuming less animal products and processed and refined foods. Over the span of many decades, it's the only way of eating that has a proven track record to prevent and even reverse chronic diseases and to help us avoid premature death. There's no denying that most "fad" diets make powerful claims, especially about losing weight quickly. However, because they are not "time tested", I would be hesitant before jumping on the "bandwagon." Combining plant based foods with moderate exercise and the avoidance of too much stress is the best option...if your goal is optimal health and well being. And, as an extra perk, you can reach your ideal weight...naturally.

If we can agree that our health is at least as important as our wealth, education and career, shouldn't we at least make enough effort to insure that we're healthy enough to fully enjoy our wealth, education and career... and our lives? Makes sense to me.

2

OUR BODY'S HEALING POWERS

"Everyone has a doctor in him or her; we just have to help it in it's work.
The natural healing force within each one of us is the greatest force in getting well."

Hippocrates 460 - 370 B.C.

FIBER:
A DISEASE FIGHTING POWERHOUSE

One of the nutrients that plants have is fiber. It is to plants what bones are to animals. The fiber is found within the plant's cell walls and it's what keeps them erect, strong and growing upwards, towards the sun. So, why is fiber so important for us humans? We've all heard that fiber is good for digestion, regularity and that it helps relieve constipation. But is that all that fiber can do for us? I remember that my mother used to take a Metamucil fiber supplement daily, a laxative made from the

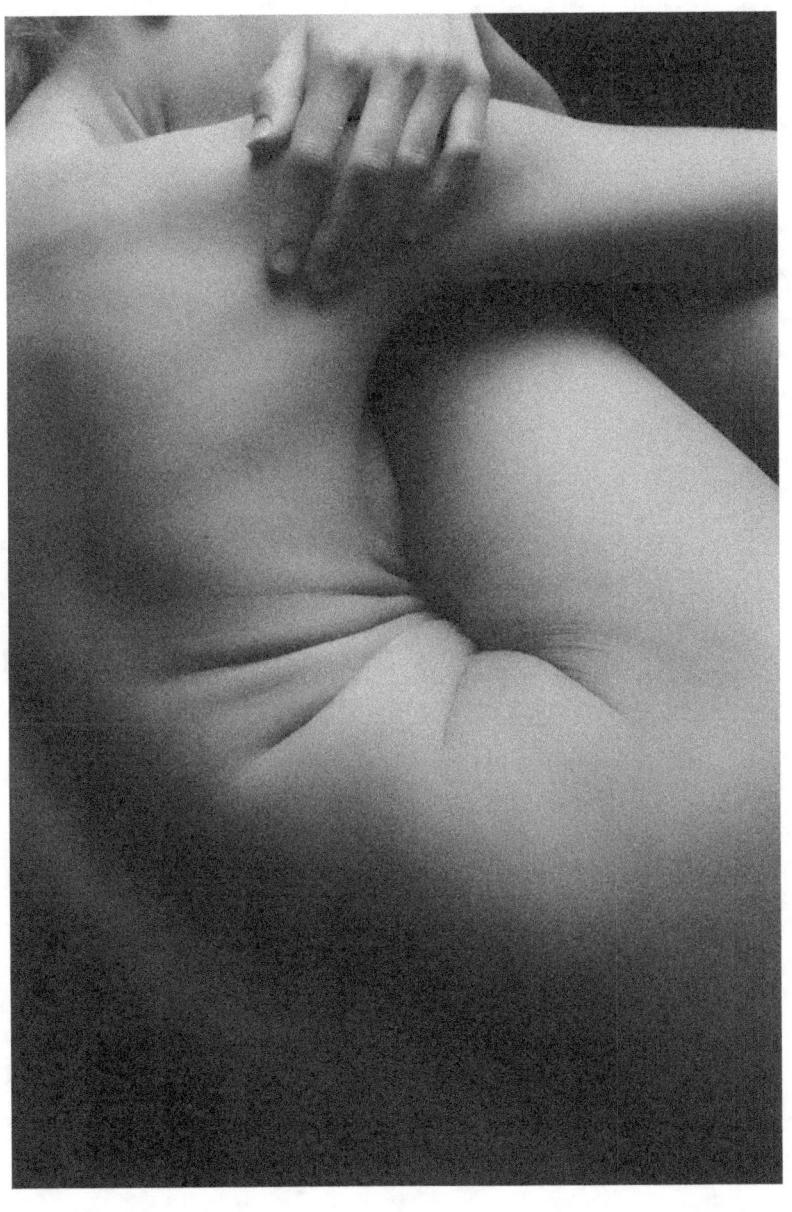

Psyllium plant and would even sprinkle some bran flakes on a piece of white toast, as an extra added fiber touch. Yet, despite that, she remained constipated throughout most of her adult years. Needless to say, fiber rich foods themselves were never an important part of her diet.

It's important to understand that animal products such as meat, dairy and eggs don't contain fiber, so we need to get it from plant foods and, if we don't get enough fiber in our diet, we could eventually experience the consequences of fiber deficiency. Yes, we often hear about vitamin and mineral deficiency and that's why we take supplements but…who tells us about fiber deficiency? According to Dr. Michael Greger in his book "How Not to Die", *"ONLY 3% OF AMERICANS MAY REACH THE RECOMMENDED MINIMUM DAILY INTAKE OF FIBER, MAKING IT ONE OF THE MOST WIDESPREAD NUTRIENT DEFICIENCIES IN THE UNITED STATES."* I would even include people, wherever they live, who consume the Standard American Diet (SAD) of meat, dairy, eggs and refined and processed foods.

HERE'S THE LOWDOWN ON FIBER:

There are two types of dietary fiber—soluble and insoluble. Soluble fiber dissolves in water and is found in a variety of fruits, vegetables, legumes, and grains. It cuts cholesterol, adds to your feeling of fullness, and slows the release of sugars from food into the blood. These actions reduce your risk for health problems including heart disease, obesity, and diabetes. Good sources of soluble fiber are oats, oat bran, oatmeal, apples,

citrus fruits, strawberries, dried beans, barley, rye flour, potatoes, raw cabbage, and pasta.

On the other hand, insoluble fiber does not dissolve in
water and is found in grain brans, fruit pulp, and vegetable
peels and skins. It is the type of fiber most strongly linked to
cancer protection and improved waste removal. Good sources
of insoluble fiber are wheat bran, whole wheat products, cereals made from bran or shredded wheat, crunchy vegetables,
barley, grains, whole wheat pasta, and rye flour.

Breaking Down Fiber: Soluble vs. Insoluble

Soluble	Insoluble
Oatmeal/oat bran	Whole-wheat breads
Nuts and seeds	Barley
Dried peas	Couscous
Beans	Brown rice
Lentils	Wheat bran
Apples	Carrots
Pears	Zucchini
Strawberries	Celery
Blueberries	Whole grain cereals

BESIDES RELIEVING CONSTIPATION,RECENT STUDIES ASSOCIATE THE FOLLOWING WITH A DIET RICH IN FIBER:

- Promotes natural weight loss – Since fiber has zero calories and is made of indigestible plant roughage, it fills
you up and curbs your appetite for extended periods.

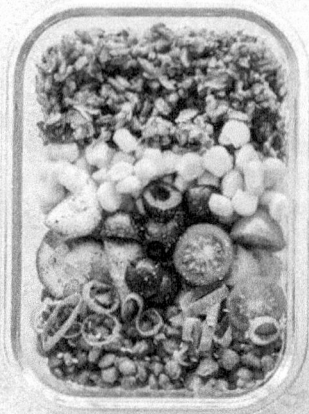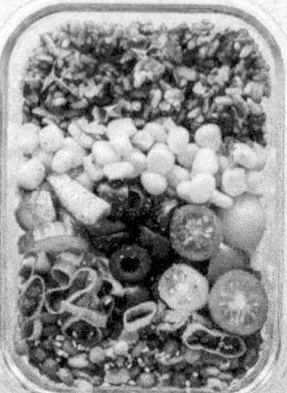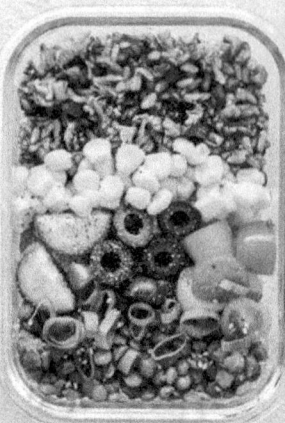

- Because it is basically undigested, fiber absorbs nasty chemicals and contaminants that might be carcinogenic and could otherwise find their way into our intestines and cause cancer.
- Prevents hemorrhoids caused by excessive straining from constipation.
- Helps to prevent colorectal cancer – For years, studies have pointed to the fact that increased fiber intake decreases the risk of colorectal cancer. This protective effect may be due to fiber's tendency to add bulk to your digestive system, shortening the amount of time that wastes travel through the colon.
- Helps to avoid diverticulosis by allowing the smooth passage of waste through the intestines.

- Reduces the risk of Type 2 Diabetes by slowing down the rate of glucose absorption and by lowering insulin levels.
- Lowers risk for arthritis by lowering inflammatory compounds in the blood.
- A high fiber diet is good for the lungs – Protects lung function, according to a study published online in the Annals of the American Thoracic Society. Those who consumed more than 17 grams of fiber per day from fruits, vegetables, and legumes had better lung health, compared with those who consumed the least.
- Fiber produces "good" gut bacteria and thus minimizes the need for probiotics.

Just as it is with vitamins and minerals, it is much healthier to choose fiber-rich foods over fiber supplements. For example, in order to get the full range of cancer-fighting phytochemicals ("phyto" means plant so phytochemicals are simply plant- compounds), we should eat whole fruits, vegetables, legumes, and grains.

TIPS FOR INCREASING FIBER IN YOUR DIET

- Choose products that are minimally processed, like whole-wheat bread instead of white bread, brown rice instead of white rice and whole wheat pasta instead of refined pasta.
- Whenever possible, do not remove the fiber-rich peels and skins of fruits and vegetables. Just be sure to wash them thoroughly before eating.

- Plan each of your meals to include whole grains, fruits, vegetables, and legumes.
- To avoid intestinal discomfort when increasing fiber intake, it is best to increase gradually and drink plenty of water.
- Snack on baby carrots, apples, strawberries, oranges, and other fiber-rich fruits and vegetables.
- Top your breakfast cereals with dried fruits like raisins or dates, or fresh fruits like strawberries or peaches.
- Sprinkle garbanzo beans or peas on your salad.
- Add a handful of grated carrots to spaghetti sauce.
- Add milled flax seeds and chia seed to fresh fruit and vegetable salads.

IF OUR TASTE BUDS COULD TALK

As a teenager, in high school, I remember an experiment in the biology class with Ritz Crackers. We were studying about the importance and role of enzymes in the digestive process. Our teacher (I don't remember his name) went around the room, passing out one cracker to each student and asking us to put it in our mouths. "What do you taste?" Everyone blurted out "Salt!" He then told us to start chewing, without swallowing, for 30 seconds. "What do you taste now?" "Sweet!" We then learned that the Ritz crackers were made from wheat, a carbohydrate, and that the enzyme Amylase, produced by the salivary glands, converted the carbohydrates (starches) into sugar, which would eventually be delivered into our muscles and liver cells...to be used as energy.

What we were told then, and what I now find very interesting, is that carnivores do not have amylase in their saliva, which strongly suggests that they do not tolerate carbohydrates. Also, carnivores, unlike us humans, don't have taste buds for sweet and that's why, if given the choice, they won't generally eat sweet foods. In fact, it could make them sick. Check this out with your cat. On the other hand, omnivores, such as our pet dog, can eat sweets, and herbivores…love sweet foods. Because of this abundance of Amylase in human saliva, and the absence of it in a carnivore's saliva, we can conclude that today's humans have evolved, both biologically and chemically, to the point where they thrive on foods rich in carbohydrates (i.e., whole grains and cereals, vegetables, fruits, nuts and seeds). And, if this is true, then maybe it would be a good idea to re-think whether or not the ever popular low carb diet is actually good for our health. Case in point: The Standard American Diet (SAD), which is a low carb diet, is consumed in populations that have the highest incidence of chronic diseases (i.e., heart cancer, type 2 diabetes, osteoporosis, rheumatoid arthritis, alzheimers).

To expand on this…since the human tongue thrives on the taste of sweet, salty and fat (front of the tongue) and less on bitter and sour (back of the tongue), why are we so enamored about the taste of meat?

Carnivores and omnivores usually eat raw meat. We humans don't. We cook our meat. And yet, I don't think most of us really enjoy plain boiled meat or chicken. It's too bland. What we do enjoy, however, is our meat, when it's fried (fat), salted or sweetened with sauces, spices and gravies. In other words, it's not the meat itself that makes us salivate. It's what we add to it that gives it that special taste. And, if it's the big 3 (salt, sweet and fat) that entices our tongues, then isn't it at all possible that by adding those same flavors to grains, cereals, vegetables, fruits and nuts, we could create extremely tasty meals. And that is exactly what happens!! The problem is that we've been programmed for so long that plant based foods cannot be tasty. When I order vegan food, on a flight, the stewardess almost always brings me this ridiculous plate of boiled and overcooked, insipid vegetables.

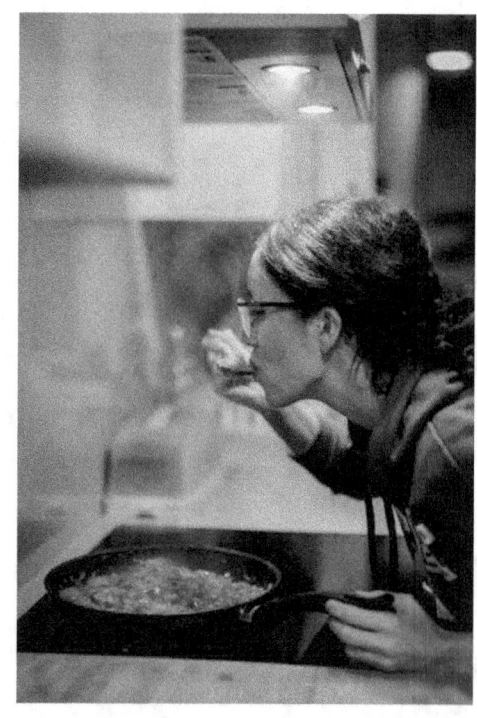

I would be much healthier if I didn't have taste buds

All it takes is a little imagination and an understanding, on the part of any cook, that many of the same flavors that are used to give taste to meats can also be used with grains and vegetables. Often, people ask me, "What will I eat?" I tell them that, besides recipe books, there are literally thousands of wonderful vegan recipes on the internet (just write vegan recipes and "click." In fact, if you write a list the ingredients you have in your cupboard, recipes using those specific ingredients will pop up on you screen.

This is also the case with dairy which, just like meat, lacks carbohydrates. Milk, cheese, butter and ice cream are loaded, in distinct proportions, with fat, salt and sugar…among other added ingredients to stimulate our taste buds. That's why we crave them.

So, if you're willing to accept the fact that we homo sapiens are designed for carbohydrates and that whole carbs are healthy for us, because they are our fountain of energy and our only source of fiber, anti-oxidants and phytonutrients… I guarantee that your taste buds will concur… and your body will reward you with optimal health.

HOW CAN WE PREVENT BREAST AND PROSTATE CANCER?

One of my pet peeves is listening to people or reading articles that claim that getting a chronic disease is a natural part of ageing. Even doctors tell us that. If we believe that statement, then we are convincing ourselves that getting a chronic disease is inevitable and there's not much we can do to prevent it.

After all, we have to die of something, right? Unfortunately, it abdicates us from the responsibility of finding out how to best take care of ourselves. It leaves us off the hook. To me that's very sad because I've learned that there are indeed things we can do, not only to help us to recover from chronic diseases but how to actually avoid them in the first place.

For young people it's critical to understand that chronic diseases don't just appear out of nowhere. We don't just get hardening of the arteries or breast or prostate cancer or type 2 diabetes. As I mentioned in my article on breast cancer, you don't all of a sudden get breast cancer. It's a process that normally develops over a period of decades. The question is, what started the process in the first place? Once we know that then the second question is…What can we could do to prevent the process from beginning in the first place? Although the cause – effect information does show the connection between environmental factors and cancer, there is extensive research based evidence showing that certain components of the Standard American Diet (aka the western diet), such as animal fat, animal protein and cholesterol are believed to initiate and promote cancer.

WHAT ABOUT HORMONES?

Years ago, my wife underwent hormone "replacement" therapy for menopausal symptoms and I remember the doctor's warning that 5 years of this therapy should be the limit, since there was already a connection between the therapy and cancer. I even checked out the manufacturer's website, where I found a

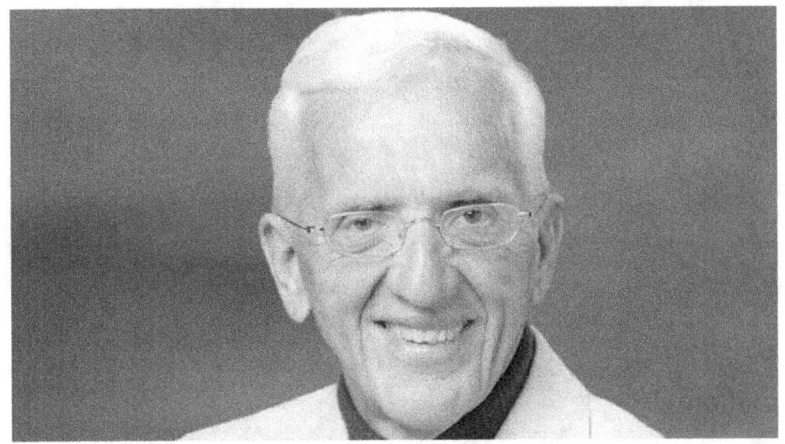

T. Colin Campbell, Ph.D
Nutritional biochemist

long list of warnings about breast cancer, uterine cancer, heart attacks, etc.

Dr. T. Colin Campbell's "CHINA STUDY" was the culmination of a 20 year partnership between Cornell University, Oxford University and the Chinese Academy of Preventive Medicine. It has sold over 2 million copies and is considered the most comprehensive study of health and nutrition ever conducted. The study resulted in more than 8,000 statistically significant associations between lifestyle, diet and disease.

One of the findings from the study linked estrogen hormone levels with breast cancer rates. Dr. Campbell states:

"This idea that breast cancer is centered on estrogen hormone exposure is profound because diet plays an important role in establishing estrogen

exposure. This suggests that the risk of breast cancer is preventable if we eat foods that will keep estrogen levels under control. The sad truth is that most women simply are not aware of this evidence. If this information were properly reported by responsible and credible public health agencies, I suspect that many more young women might be taking very real, very effective steps to avoid this awful disease."

Research shows that eating lots of fiber rich foods (only found in plants) helps to eliminate excess estrogen from the body.

To support this, Dr. Neal Barnard, President of the Physicians Committee for Responsible Medicine writes:

"Every minute of every day, your liver filters your blood, removing toxins and anything else that your body needs to get rid of. That includes excess hormones. The liver sends these unwanted compounds through a

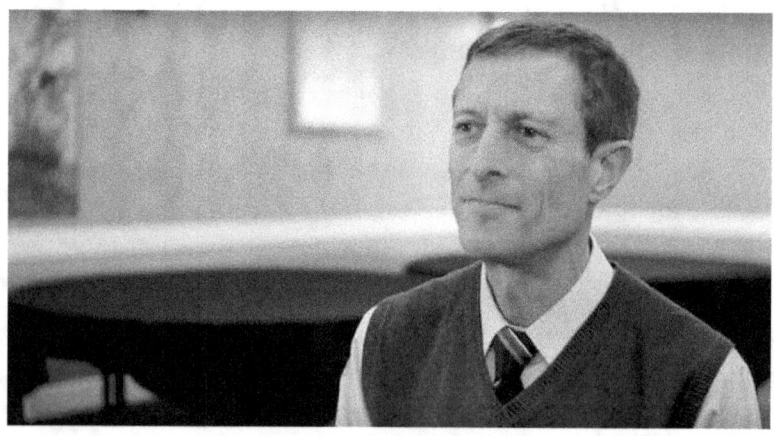

Neal Barbard, M. D.
Researcher on diet & health

narrow tube called the bile duct into your intestinal tract. There, fiber (plant roughage) soaks them up and carries them out of the body with the wastes."

HORMONES, COW'S MILK and CANCER

A hormone is a natural chemical that our body produces that has specific functions. They are chemical messengers that tell the cells and organs what to do. (i.e., the Insulin hormone from the pancreas regulates blood sugar while adrenaline, produced by the adrenal glands, can regulate heart rate, give is extra strength, etc.). The body produces hormones according to it's needs. Estrogen is a hormone that is produced within a woman's body and is responsible for breast development among other bodily functions. The body normally produces the amount it needs.

According to Dr. Michael Greger, author of the NY Times Best Seller "HOW NOT TO DIE":

"Mother nature designed cow's milk to put a few hundred pounds on a baby calf within a few months. A lifetime of human exposure to these growth factors in milk may help explain the connections found between dairy consumption and certain cancers. Leading Harvard University nutrition experts have expressed concern that the hormones in dairy products and other growth factors could stimulate the growth of hormone sensitive tumors."

Cow's produce enough estrogen to meet their own needs and the level increases when they are pregnant. When we consume milk and dairy products we are consuming a cow's estrogens among the other hormones that a cow naturally produces. Dairy and cheesemakers don't do anything to remove the hormones. In fact, farmers often inject extra hormones into cows to fatten them and to increase milk production. One example is Bovine Growth Hormone which is a GMO created in 1994 by Monsanto. It has resulted in so many health problems among cows, especially infections, that antibiotics are necessary to counter the problem (we consume those too). As a result, bovine growth hormone is now banned in Canada, the European Union, Australia, New Zealand, Japan and Israel. Unfortunately, it's still being used on many U.S. dairy farms.

Since prostate cancer is considered the male equivalent of breast cancer the connection between milk and dairy and prostate cancer is similar…as revealed in many studies. Yet, for me the studies of populations of people worldwide are some of the most convincing. Prostate cancer is rare in parts of the world where people eat a low- fat, nearly-vegetarian diet. For example, there is 120 times less incidence of prostate cancer in China compared to men in the United States. However, as these populations of Chinese people change to the Western diet, their risk increases proportionally.

As I mentioned at the beginning of this post it's very important for both men and women, of all ages, to grasp the significance of the fact that the journey of chronic diseases often begins at an early age…even in childhood. So, if living healthy and to a ripe old age is important to us, we should consider substituting a lot more healthy plant based foods into our diet in place of meat and dairy.

9 SECRETS TO A LONGER AND HEALTHIER LIFE

Sometimes I would ask people, "would you like to live to 100?" The answers would summon approximately 50% yeses and 50% noes. My wife, Delia always gives it an emphatic NO! Why? "Well, she replies, just look at what people look like when they get old." I do remind that when she was 60, her age limit goal was 70. Now she's in her 70s and her goal has jumped to "somewhere in the 80s." When asked why she updates her goals, she says, "well, as long as I feel well, I'd like to keep on going." In other words, when it comes down to it, I think that, as with other living species, we don't want to die. We want to live as long as possible...as long as we're feeling healthy and enjoying our life.

In 2008, National Geographic explorer Dan Buettner, and his team, began searching for the world's healthiest, happiest and longest living people (100+ years). The result was his NY Times Best Seller "The Blue Zones." From his research and interviews during the next two years he came upon 5 population groups, which he named the "Blue Zones." With the hope that we can benefit from what he discovered, the author shares with us the keys to their long and healthy life.

In Dan Buettner's own words:
For 30 years, my life's work has been identifying and then studying extraordinary populations around the world and unlocking their secrets to longevity and happiness.

Life expectancy of an American born today averages 78.2 years. But this year, over 70,000 Americans have reached their

100th birthday. What are they doing that the average American isn't (or won't?).

To answer the question, we teamed up with National Geographic to find the world's longest-lived people and study them. We knew most of the answers lied within their lifestyle and environment (The Danish Twin Study established that only about 20% of how long the average person lives is determined by genes.). Then we worked with a team of demographers to find pockets of people around the world with the highest life

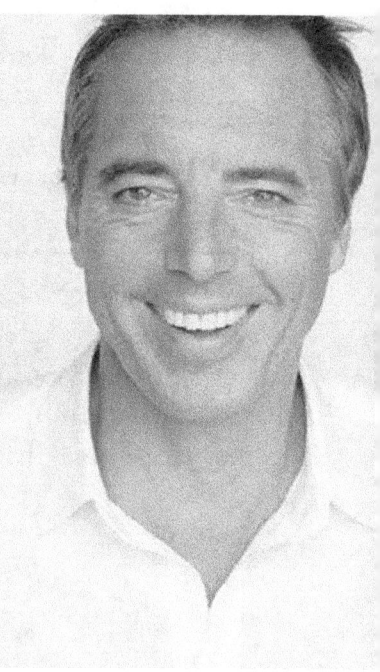

Dan Buettner

expectancy, or with the highest proportions of people who reach age 100. People in these "Blue Zones" regions not just live longer, but they live better. Besides having a large number of centenarians, people in these areas remain active into their 80s and 90s and do not suffer from the chronic diseases common in most parts of the industrialized world.

WE FOUND FIVE PLACES THAT MET OUR CRITERIA:

- Barbagia region of Sardinia – Mountainous highlands of inner Sardinia with the world's highest concentration of male centenarians.
- Ikaria, Greece – Aegean Island with one of the world's lowest rates of middle age mortality and the lowest rates of dementia.
- Nicoya Peninsula, Costa Rica – World's lowest rates of middle age mortality, second highest concentration of male centenarians.
- Seventh Day Adventists – Highest concentration is around Loma Linda, California. They live 10 years longer than their North American counterparts.
- Okinawa, Japan – Females over 70 are the longest-lived population in the world.

We then assembled a team of medical researchers, anthropologists, demographers, and epidemiologists to search for evidence-based common denominators among all places.

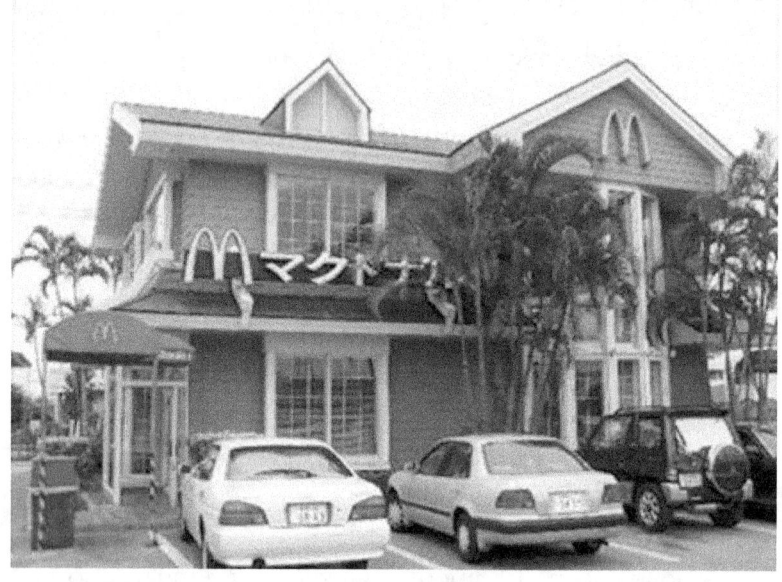

Hanby Town, Okinawa

WE FOUND 9:

1 **Move naturally throughout the day.** Centenarians live in environments that constantly nudge them into moving without thinking about it.

2 Have and cultivate **a strong sense of purpose.** "Why do I wake up in the morning."

3 **Downshift** every day to relieve stress (i.e., meditation, exercise, napping).

4 **80% Rule:** Stop eating when you are 80 percent full.

5 **Plant Slant:** Beans (fava, black, soy and lentils), whole grains, veggies, and fruit are the cornerstone of

centenarian diets. Meat is rarely eaten (average 5 times a month and in small portions (3-4 oz.).

6   **Wine:** Enjoy wine and alcohol moderately with friends and/or food.

7   **Belong:** Be part of a faith-based community or organization. Denomination doesn't matter.

8   **Love Ones First:** Have close friends and strong family connections Successful centenarians in the Blue Zones put their families first. This means keeping aging parents and grandparents nearby or in the home (It lowers disease and mortality rates of children in the home too.). They commit to a life partner (which can add up to 3 years of life expectancy) and invest in their children with time and love (They'll be more likely to care for you when the time comes).

9   **Right Tribe:** Cultivate close friends and strong social networks. The world's longest lived people chose—or were born into—social circles that supported healthy behaviors.

At the beginning of this exploration, we were interested in figuring out if DNA had anything to do with the exceptional health and longevity in these regions. What we learned was that it's not DNA and it's not geography. As the Western-influenced lifestyle and diet come in, these "Blue Zones" regions are dying out. The reason most of these places had such incredible health outcomes was partially because they were isolated, geographically, from the rest of the world. It took a while for fast food, processed food, and large quantities of meat to infiltrate their diets. But as we see in Okinawa, Japan, the newer generation has a more modern lifestyle and eat a more Western-pattern diet. And now they are starting to have the health problems of the Western world. Their geographic location hasn't changed—their lifestyle has.

So, are you ready to take the next step?
For health seekers, interested in including all or some of these 9 "common denominators", into their lifestyle, I suggest first making a "mental" checklist of 1) which ones we are presently including into our lifestyle, 2) which ones we should be including and 3) which ones cannot be included, for whatever reason. For example, move naturally throughout the day might not be feasible for someone having to sit at a desk for 8 hours.

Once that's done then you can rank these common denominators according to a hierarchy based on what is important to you. For example, making a change to a more plant based diet, if you're not doing that now (Plant Slant), is probably more important for your health, than whether or not you're drinking wine.

My personal hierarchy of importance would be: 1) Plant Slant, 2) Relieve Stress, 3) Strong sense of Purpose, 4) Belong, 5) Move Naturally, 6) Love ones First, 7) Right Tribe, 8) 80% Rule, 9) Wine. My priority for the past 8 years has been a Whole Food Plant Based Diet (Plant Slant) + Meditation + Exercise. Now, at the ripe and healthy age of 76, I feel that it's time to dedicate more time and energy to some of the other common denominators from the Blue Zones.

What about you?

WHERE DOES THE BEST DOCTOR IN THE WORLD LIVE?

In India?
In Japan?
In China?
In the United States?
Noooooooooooooooooo!!!!!!!!!!!!

The best doctor in the world actually lives inside each one of us. The only problem is that we never think of it that way. We never make the connection. For us, the only real doctor is the external one…the one who prescribes the pills…or the surgery…or the chemo, etc.

Yet, according to **Hippocrates**, the "Father of Medicine":

Everyone has a doctor in him or her; we just have to help it in its work. The natural healing force within each one of us is the greatest force in getting well.

How good is this inner doctor?
Well…

- It's the one who heals us when we break a bone. Yes, the external doctor puts on the cast but it's the inner doctor that actually heals the bone.

- It's the one who cares for us so much that it labors 24/7 to keep us healthy. Since it labors 24/7, we don't have to make an appointment and we're not charged anything for it's service.
- It's the one that constantly fights off viral and bacterial infections…whether we're aware of it or not.
- It's the one that tells us if something is not right (with pain and discomfort) and when everything is just right, with a feeling of well being.

This list can go on and on but, what's most important is to be able to change our way of thinking and accept and be thankful that this wonderful and loving inner doctor does exist.

How can we be thankful?

By treating our bodies with respect…so that it keeps us well and heals us when we are sick.

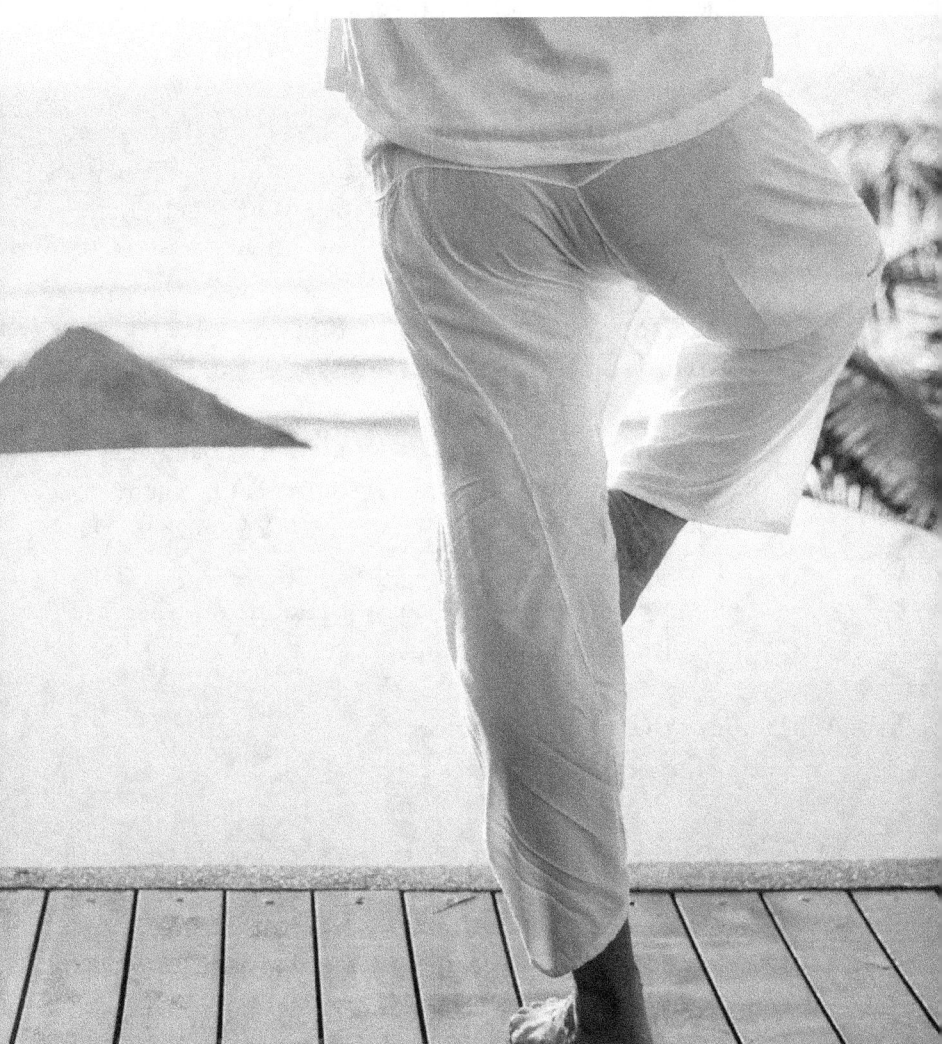

How can we treat our bodies with respect?
Well, after 76 years of life on this planet, 34 on the Standard American Diet of mostly meat, dairy and eggs, 32 as a vegetarian and the last 8 as a whole food vegan I have a few suggestions, based on things that I have learned and practice:

- What's most important is sticking, as close as possible, to a whole food plant based regimen (grains, cereals, fruits, vegetables, nuts and seeds). Your inner doctor will thank you for making it's work a lot easier.
- Exercise at least 5 days a week. I take brisk 40 minute walks and go to the gym 2 or 3 times a week.
- Avoid, as much as possible, excess stress and pressure. I've been practicing meditation for more than 40 years and it helps me stay centered and look at daily occurrences and problems from a distance. With regards to feeling pressure, it's a good idea to detect where the pressure is coming from because of the tendency to put pressure on ourselves when we shouldn't or, when the pressure should be on someone else…not ourselves.

What about the external doctors?
Well, Hippocrates then goes on to say:

The greatest medicine of all is teaching people how not to need it.

In other words, the main role of a "good" external doctor is to work hand and hand with our inner doctor, to help our bodies maintain optimum health and well being and, if we do get sick, to help our bodies to cure itself. When we forget about our inner doctor, then we put ourselves at the mercy of the external doctor and his or her decisions, whatever they may be. Unfortunately, as in most cases what doctors are most interested in is treating the symptoms instead of decease prevention and reversal. This is what the best doctor in the world is up against.

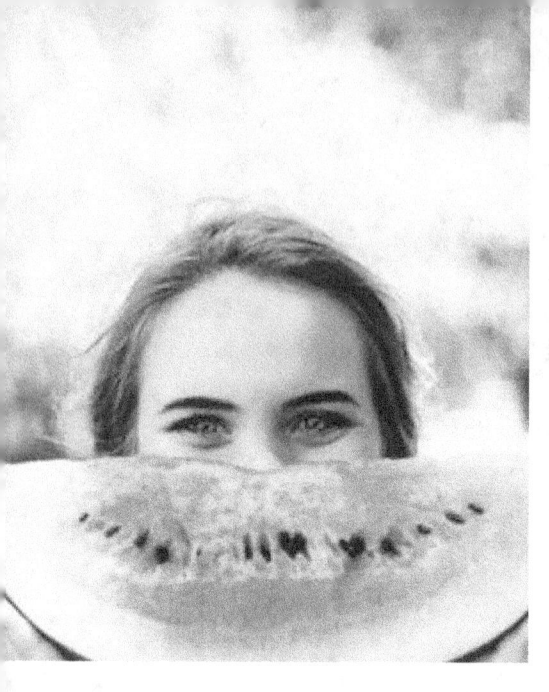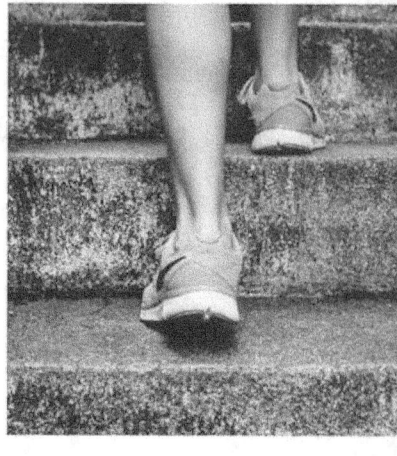

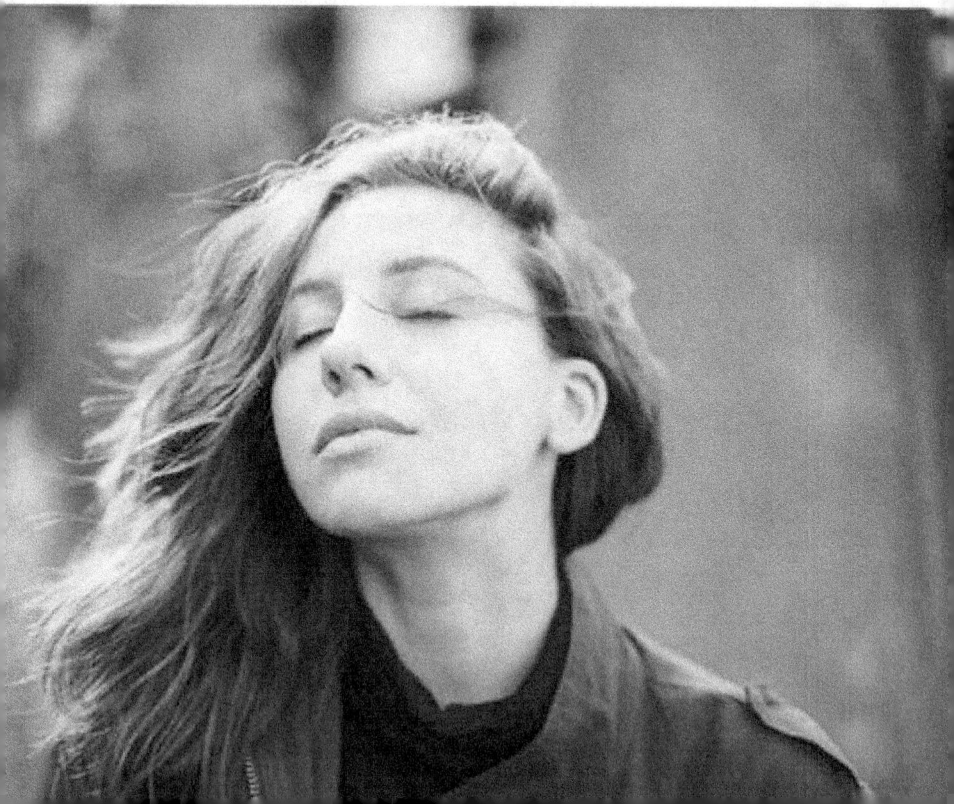

3

REFUTING THE SACRED COWS OF NUTRITION

"The problem is we are not eating food anymore.
We are eating food like products."
Dr. Alejandro Jünger,
author of the "Clean Program"

CHALLENGING BELIEFS WITH "KNOWLEDGE"

About three months ago I began to promote some of my nutrition posts on my Facebook page without knowing what results it would bring. I've been pleasantly surprised about the number of people who have had the opportunity to read what I have to say…more than 60,000 and counting. People have responded in many different ways to the information that I'm sharing, but what has really caught my attention are the number of people who have responded because their beliefs on nutrition have been challenged… beliefs that are deep rooted. To accept that one's beliefs maybe wrong is not easy for most people…it's just not a comfortable feeling. It requires a person to be

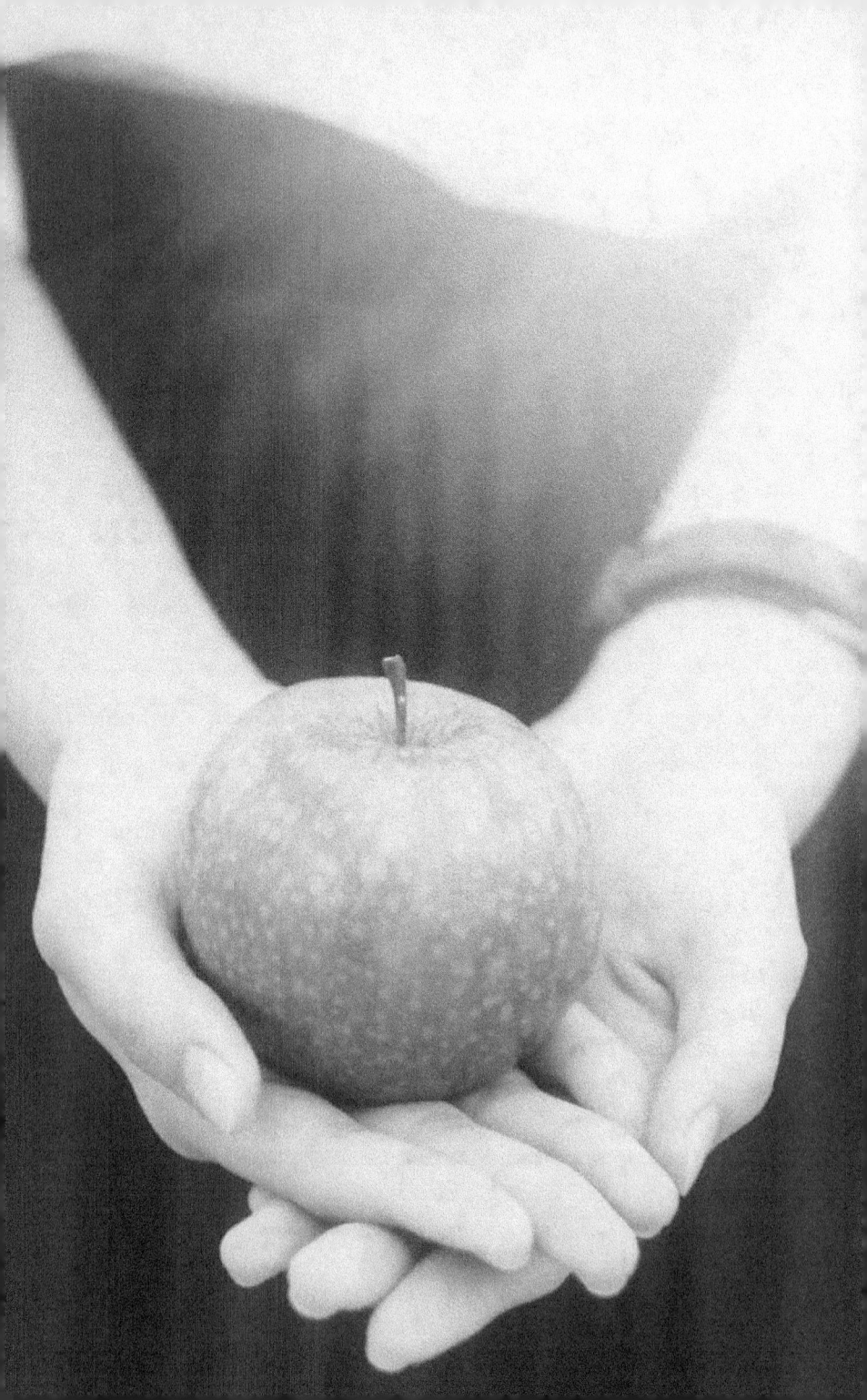

open to seeing things in a new light and that's not so simple, especially with regards to beliefs that we have been cherishing for a long time…even since early childhood. Some of these beliefs about nutrition are so strong that they have actually become part of our culture. To challenge that is not an easy task. Yet, because of my understanding and knowledge of the power and benefits of whole food vegan nutrition and it's capacity to prevent and even reverse chronic diseases…I'm more than willing to accept the challenge.

What's very important for me is that what I write makes sense to the reader…it's as simple as that. There is so much conflicting information on nutrition out there the question is, how can we discern what is true and what is false? Yet, I am convinced that when something makes sense to us it goes beyond our thought process. It touches us a little deeper and as a result, we understand something that we didn't understand before.

So, my goal is to make sense… to you the reader.

Once a new idea makes sense then a belief can become "knowing." That comes about when we decide to make a change and begin to experience improvement to our health. Without that "knowing" we just continue believing.

As a first step for anyone who would like to learn a new approach to nutrition, one that make sense, I suggest watching the wonderful and powerful documentary "Forks over Knives" (Tenedores contra Cuchillos), It's available for free on Netflix and youtube and has Spanish subtitles. The documentary is fact based and includes interviews with reknowned doctors, nutritionists and experts in the field of nutrition.

As a follow up, another impacting video is "What the Health", also available with Spanish subtitles on Netflix and youtube. It takes a different approach to nutrition by confronting and exposing the powerful industries of Agriculture and Dairy as well as highly respected organizations such as the American Heart Association, the American Diabetes Association and the American Cancer Society.

SO, WHERE DO YOU GET YOUR PROTEIN FROM?

I can't remember how many times I've been asked that question. I do enjoy answering it, although **I really can't understand why people still ask it.** As I flex my biceps, my first response is, "Look at me! I'm 77 years old and haven't eaten meat since 1976. Do I look sick, lethargic or in pain? "After all these meatless decades, I must have a protein deficiency... right?"

Unfortunately, sometimes that's not proof enough for certain people...so I advance to response #2:

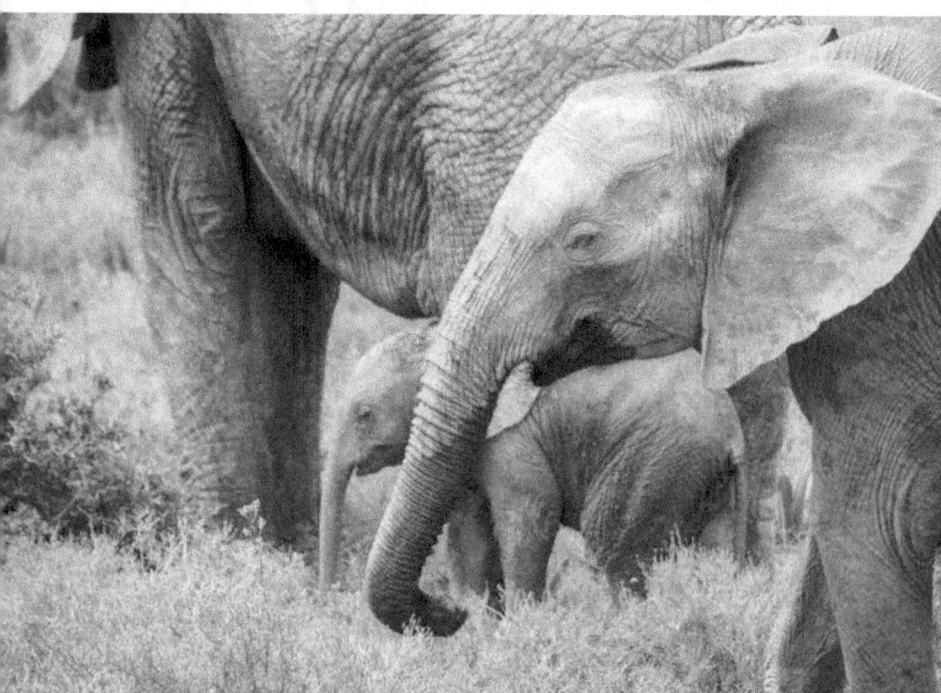

"What are 2 things elephants, gorillas, rhinoceri, hippos, water buffalos and the now extinct 50 ton brachiosaurus, have in common?"

First of all, I think we can agree that they are among the largest and strongest land animals to have ever roamed the earth and secondly...they are and were plant eaters! So, where do they get their proteins from? Plants. If these animals can thrive on plant based foods...why can't humans, with our relatively tiny bodies, thrive on plants as well? Doesn't it make sense? Also, cows get their protein from plants and we believe that we need to get our protein from killing and eating the cows. Why not get it direct from the source? It not only saves a cow, a chicken or a pig's life, it's also healthier because plants 1) don't come with the burdens of cholesterol and saturated fats that lead to health problems, while they 2) provide us with the disease preventing benefits of fiber, anti-oxidants and phytonutrients...which all happen to be lacking in meat.

NOT CONVINCED YET?

Well, as a last resort to the remaining deniers, I move on to my third and last response:

Some of the world's elite athletes are turning to plant based nutrition and, as a result, are experiencing improved performances by boosting blood flow and oxygenations of their muscles while taking advantage of a vegan diet's anti-inflammatory effect to speed their post workout recovery. To name a few:

Tom Brady – Quarterback of the New England Patriots. At the age of 40 is performing as well as ever and believes he can continue to play at this level for several more years.

Serena and Venus Williams – Two of the greatest tennis players of all time…still playing after 20 years.

Lionel Messi – Considered one of history's greatest soccer players.

Carl Lewis – Winner of 10 Olympic Gold Medals during the 1990s.

Kyrie Irving – NBA 2012 rookie of the year and 2014 All-Star MVP.

Lewis Hamilton – four time winner of the Formula One World Drivers'Championship.

Meagan Duhamel – figure skating gold medalist at the 2018 olympics. **Patrik Baboumian** – powerlifter and named Germany's strongest man. **Scott Jurek** – considered the greatest ultra-marathoner of modern times.

Tia Blanco – Open Women's World Surfing Champion two consecutive years.

Steph Davis – one of the greatest female rock climbers in the world.

David "hayemaker" Haye – Former two time heavyweight boxing champion To see dozens more elite vegan athletes, check out: greatveganathletes.com

There's another area that "all of the above" have in common and that is **"staying active."** In the wild, the animals are constantly moving around (not so in zoos). There are no couch potatoes in the jungle. Same with athletes…practice, practice, practice. For me, it's going to the gym and going on daily walks and remembering to get off my butt, by tearing myself away from the computer… ever so often.

CONCLUSION:

The myth that we have believed in for so long (since childhood), regarding meat being the best form of protein for us humans, has never been true. Yes, meat provides complete proteins, as do plants, but it's not the healthiest source….for your heart, your waistline, your overall health. So, based upon the above information, I suggest replacing meat with plant options such as beans, tofu, lentils, chickpeas, quinoa, chia, peanuts, almonds, kale, etc. Even gradual replacement is a good start because a **"little bit of something is better than a lot of nothing."** And don't worry whether you're getting enough protein because, as long as you eat a variety of plant based foods, over time, and don't starve yourself, you'll never be protein deficient.

TRUTHS ABOUT MILK AND CHEESE
PART 1

An esoteric teacher, George Gurdjieff, once said:

"Man is made in such a way that he is never so attached to anything as he is to his suffering."

As true as that may be, in order to prove a point, I made a slight change…

Man is made in such a way that he is never so attached to anything as he is to his… Cheese.

Whenever I talk with someone about the option of a vegan diet, what the great majority expresses is that they can give up meat but to give up cheese, and in general, dairy products, would be a major challenge. Meat…not so hard. Dairy…hard.

For me it was no different. I became a vegetarian in 1976, but until 8 years ago, I found it difficult to sacrifice my cheese. My brother, who has been following a vegan lifestyle for 12 years and is a healthy, energetic and productive individual at the age of 82, suggested I read up on dairy products. So I did. What I found from my reading and watching videos was that, besides the high saturated fat, cholesterol and hormone content, another major concern with milk and dairy is…**calcium**.

If you ask the average person why is milk so important? The answer will almost inadvertently be calcium.

So, what about the calcium in cows milk?

The problem is not the calcium…there's plenty of that in milk and dairy products. The problem is the acidity in the animal protein found in all dairy products.

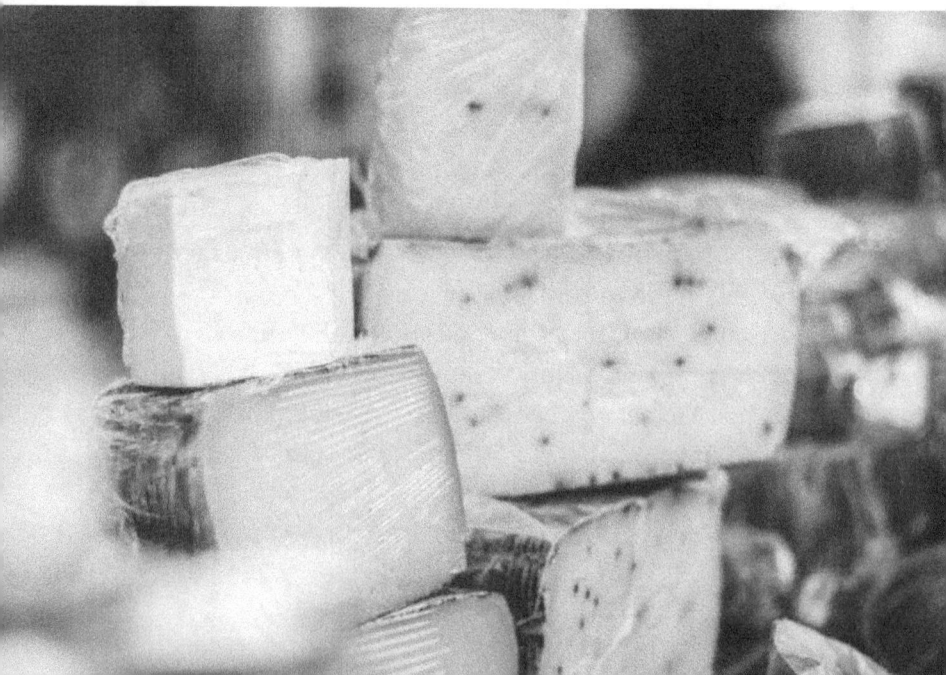

According to Vivian Goldschmidt, MA, founder of the Save Institute, The Save Our Bones Program and an expert on treating osteoporosis, naturally:

Milk depletes the calcium from your bones.

"The milk myth has spread around the world based on the flawed belief that this protein and calcium-rich drink is essential to support good overall health and bone health in particular at any age. It is easy to understand that the confusion about milk's imaginary benefits stems from the fact that it contains calcium – around 300 mg per cup.

But many scientific studies have shown an assortment of detrimental health effects directly linked to milk consumption. And the most surprising link is that not only do we barely absorb the calcium in cow's milk (especially if pasteurized), but to make matters worse, it actually increases calcium loss from the bones. What an irony this is!

Here's how it happens. Like all animal protein, milk acidifies the body pH which in turn triggers a biological correction. You see, calcium is an excellent acid neutralizer and the biggest storage of calcium in the body is – you guessed it… in the bones. So the very same calcium that our bones need to stay strong is utilized to neutralize the acidifying effect of milk. Once calcium is pulled out of the bones, it leaves the body via the urine, so that the surprising net result after this is an actual calcium deficit.

Knowing this, you'll understand why statistics show that countries with the lowest consumption of dairy products also have the lowest fracture incidence in their population.

But the sad truth is that most mainstream health practitioners ignore these proven facts. I know it firsthand because when I was diagnosed with osteoporosis, my doctor recommended that I drink lots of milk in addition to taking Fosamax."

Dr. Joel Fuhrman, author of "Eat to Live", and one of my wise doctors, writes:

"Hip fractures and osteoporosis are more frequent in populations in which dairy products are commonly consumed and calcium intakes are commonly high. For example, American women drink thirty to thirty two times as much cow's milk as New Guineans, yet suffer forty-seven times as many broken hips. A multi-country analysis of hip fracture incidence and dairy product consumption found that milk consumption has a high statistical association with higher rates of hip fractures."

SINCE BIRTH WE WERE TOLD
"DRINK MORE MILK,
GET STRONG BONES"

COUNTRIES WITH THE HIGHEST CONSUPTION OF MILK	COUNTRIES WITH THE HIGHEST RATE OF OSTEOPOROSIS
US	US
ENGLAND	ENGLAND
SWEDEN	SWEDEN
FINLAND	FINLAND

Dr. John McDougall, another wise doctor, adds:

"All minerals, including calcium, come originally from the ground and enter animals through plants. Which means plants are loaded with calcium, iron, zinc, copper, etc., and the more plants you eat the more minerals you acquire. The relationship between people and plants works so well that there has never been a case of dietary calcium deficiency ever reported.

To put it even more clearly: all-plant diets are sufficient to meet the needs of growing children and adults (infants need breast milk). Calcium pills have a few adverse effects like constipation and inhibition of iron absorption. The most serious mistake a person can make is to believe cow's milk is a "good" and necessary source of calcium. Heart disease, cancer, type-2 diabetes, arthritis, and infectious disease are only a few of the common consequences of drinking milk from other animal species"

TRUTHS ABOUT
MILK AND CHEESE
PART 2

"It seems ridiculous that a man, in midst of his pleasures, should have to go beneath a cow…like a calf, three times a day…never weaned."

Henry David Thoreau

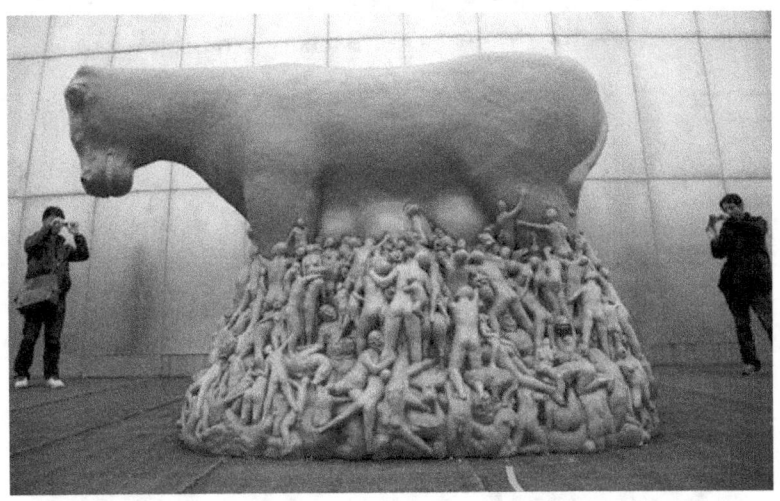

Liu Qiang

Human beings are the only animal that drinks the milk of another animal. Not only that, but as Thoreau states, it's the only adult animal in nature that was never weaned from milk. All other baby animals, at one point or another, no longer return to their mother's breasts, as nature intended it to be. Yet, we intelligent humans decided to break with nature's law and not only continue to consume milk but also process it into dairy products, such as cheese, butter, yogurt and ice cream.

HOW DID ALL THIS COME ABOUT?

Well, there was a time when humans didn't drink the milk of other animals, a time when osteoporosis and bone fractures were rare. Today, most of the world's population doesn't consume dairy (i.e., rural China, Japan, India and parts of Africa) and rarely experience osteoporosis and fractures. That's also the case with some of the world's strongest vegan animals (i.e., gorillas, elephants, rhinos, water buffalos) and numerous elite

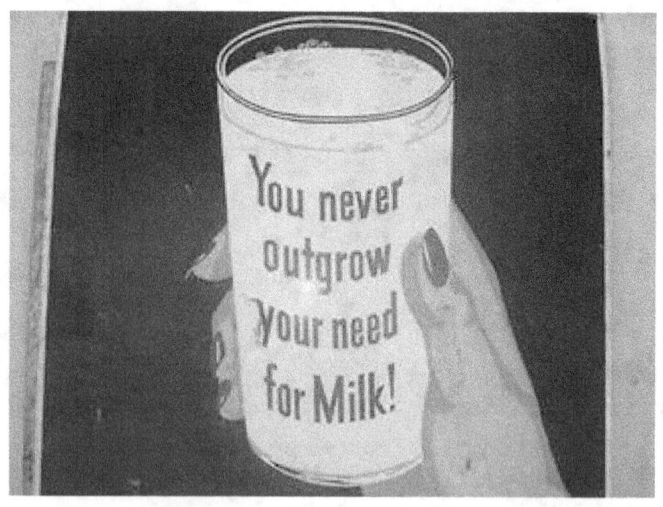

vegan athletes (i.e., Tom Brady – football, Kyrie Irving – basketball, Serena and Venus Williams – tennis, Lionel Messi – soccer, Carl Lewis – Olympics, David Haye – boxing, Scott Jurek – ultra-marathoner, Marc Danzig – martial arts, etc.).

Despite the overwhelming research evidence showing the connection between the consumption of milk and dairy and chronic diseases such as heart, cancer, diabetes 2, osteoporosis, rheumatoid arthritis, hypertension and obesity, our love affair and attachment seems to be unbreakable. For so many on the Standard American Diet, milk is still the "perfect" food, as American as "apple pie" and the "flag." The intense promotion of milk and dairy by dairy institutions has been going on since the early 1900s.

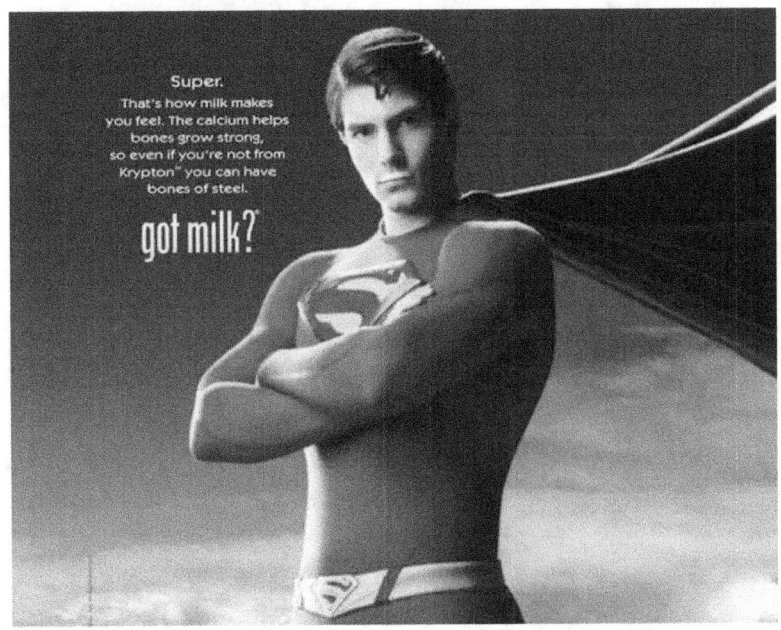

One of the first slogans I clearly remember from elementary school was *"YOU NEVER OUTGROW YOUR NEED FOR MILK."*

Whenever sales dropped marketing teams came up with new slogans such as "MILK LIFE" and the famous moustache adds…"GOT MILK?"

A fortune was spent on the "got milk" adds, promoted by many notable people in politics, sports and the entertainment industry. As a result, milk and dairy sales again skyrocketed and the industries' CEOs and investors were once again… satisfied! In the words of Jeff Manning, executive director of the California Milk Processor Board, **"This is our objective statement today: Sell More Milk. Everything that we do, every moment that I spend, gets filtered through this objective. If it doesn't sell more milk or have the potential to sell more milk, we won't do it – It's just that simple."** The Dairy Industry's prime objective is to sell as much milk and dairy products to as many people possible.

Does that sound like our health is their priority?

And if health is indeed an issue, **WHY IS IT SO DIFFICULT FOR MOST PEOPLE TO STOP CONSUMING DAIRY?**

According to Dr. Neal Barnard, author of the NY Times best seller "The Cheese Trap", nature has gifted all pregnant female animals with a substance in their milk called casomorphin. Just this word should get you thinking…morphine? Yes. It's an opiate and It's mother nature's way of making sure that the baby returns time and again to it's mother's breast. Nature is just not taking any chances! What does that mean for us humans? Well, by consuming a small dosage of a cow's casomorphin, maybe that's what keeps us coming back for more cheese…or pizza or cheeseburgers. In other words, because of the casomorphin, we've actually become addicted to cow's milk and dairy products.

AND HOW (UN)HEALTHY IS COW'S MILK?

For the calf, it's the perfect food! For humans, whether babies or grownups, it's far from perfect.

As I mentioned in a previous post, as a vegetarian I became sick at least once a year with a sore throat, a cough and/or chest congestion. Once I turned whole food vegan, I never got sick again…8 years and counting. However, at first and even though my brother Arthur tried to convince me about the benefits of whole food plant based nutrition, it was difficult to surrender my attachment to cheese. What changed everything for me and brought me some clarity was the book he insisted that I read…" The China Study", by T. Colin Campbell, PHD. With over 2 million copies sold it's considered to be the most comprehensive study of nutrition ever conducted. I consider it a must read for anyone interested in nutrition facts soundly based on research studies.

So, here are some of my conclusions from these past 2 posts as well as points to consider regarding milk and dairy… based on my own personal experience and research during these past 8 years:

- **Cow's milk is designed for calves, not humans and especially adult humans. The fat, protein and hormone content is meant to grow a cow and is way too high and therefore unhealthy for human consumption. Think about it: A cow doubles it's birth weight at 47 days. A human at 180 days**

- "Milk builds strong bones" is a myth fed to us since childhood. The calcium in milk actually has the opposite effect...leading to osteoporosis and hip fractures.
- **Since all calcium comes originally from plants, why not avoid the middle man... the cow. That's what the strongest animals do (i.e., elephant, rhinoceros, gorilla, water buffalo, hippo and even the extinct brontosaurus). A cow doesn't get it's calcium from eating another cow!!**
- Populations that don't consume dairy (i.e., rural China and Japan, India and parts of Africa) rarely suffer the chronic diseases as populations that do consume dairy.
- **Mountains of research show the connection between milk and dairy and chronic diseases such as cancer, heart disease, osteoporosis, rheumatoid arthritis, diabetes 2 and obesity. Removal of dairy from our diets has been shown to prevent and often reverse these same diseases.**
- Dairy institutions spend 100 billion dollars annually on slogans, propaganda and unsubstantiated studies to keep us confused and therefore not open to changing our diet.
- **Cheese is concentrated calories from fat that makes us overweight and obese. One cup of milk = 149 calories whereas one cup of melted cheddar = 986 calories.**
- Countries that consume the most dairy have the highest per capita incidence of osteoporosis and hip fractures (i.e., United States, United Kingdom, Australia, Sweden, Finland, Germany, etc.).

- **Cheese is arguably the most processed food on the planet (pasteurized, fermented by bacteria, coagulated with enzymes, separated into solids, salted and aged and further processed when added to pizza and casseroles).**
- In 1909 the average American ate 4 pounds of cheese per year. In 2013 the annual intake climbed to 33 pounds.
- **Cheese is loaded with salt which is added as a preservative and flavoring. Not good for our blood pressure**
- Fiber is not only important for digestion and the production of good bacteria in the gut but helps us to feel full and control our appetite. Cheese has zero fiber so that you can eat a lot of it before feel satisfied.
- **Milk is addictive because of the morphine like compound, casomorphin, found in the milk protein...casein. Cheese is even more addictive because of the added salt and fat. In other words, it's not easy for many people, to break the habit. That's the way it was for me.**

And last but not least...

- It is estimated that worldwide, ¾ of the population is lactose intolerant after childhood (Asians – 90%, African Americans – 75%, Mexican Americans – 50%). This is because, in most cases, the enzyme lactase which digests the complex sugar lactose in milk, is usually no longer produced by the body, after the age of 4. This can lead to symptoms such as headaches, cramps, gas, bloating, nausea and diarrhea. Yet, if you don't make the connection, then you could be suffering from the symptoms without knowing the real cause...trying in vain one remedy after another. This happened with my son Adán. When he was very young, every time he got a fever, he got headaches and convulsions. His eyes would role back into his head and sometimes he would become unconscious. Needless to say, It was very scary for him and us. Whenever he came down with a fever he would inevitably cry...expecting the inevitable return of the convulsions. Eventually we met a Naturopath doctor who concluded, after we told him that he would gulp down 3 or four glasses of chocolate milk every day, that Adán was lactose intolerant. End of story and convulsions as Adán hasn't tasted milk or dairy for the past 35 years. By the way, he's an extreme sports professional.

WHAT'S WRONG WITH LOW CARB DIETS?

"People like to hear good things about their bad habits."

It started years ago and continues to this day...the controversy or the conflict between low carb and high carb diets. The Standard American Diet (SAD) was, is and always will be a low carb diet and that's because it's based on the consumption of meat dairy and eggs...foods that have almost no carbohydrates. How healthy is that? Well, if you look at the results, for those on the SAD diet, you'll see that chronic diseases such as heart, cancer, type 2 diabetes, osteoporosis, Alzheimer's, etc., are not about to disappear. In fact, every year, the health situation seems to be getting worse.

Because of this poor "report card", during the past few decades, people have been looking for and experimenting with other diet options (i.e., Atkins diet – 1972 Eat Right for Your Type – 1997, Paleo Diet – 2002, South Beach Diet – 2005). Unfortunately, these options are basically just off springs of the SAD and since the SAD is not a very healthy diet, it appears to me that the main reason for people changing diets is to shed pounds in order to look better in other people's eyes and secondarily... to improve their own health. The initial weight loss does happen but at the expense of good health and wellness. Because of the high content of saturated fat and cholesterol found in meat, dairy and eggs and the lack of fiber, vitamins, minerals, antioxidants and phytonutrients which is found in plant foods, it's difficult to maintain a quick weight loss diet for more than a few weeks, without suffering the consequences. What's the result? In most cases it's a return to the original SAD, where pounds are put on again... or jump on to another diet bandwagon with the hope that this time it will work...long term. After all, there's a lot of options to choose from (Wikipedia lists more than 100 different diets). You can actually pinball from one diet to another...for the rest of your life and not get the results you want.

It's important to understand that the only healthy carbs are unprocessed ones, found in whole grains and cereals, vegetables, fruits, nuts and seeds. These healthy carbs are converted into complex sugars that provide continuous energy to our cells. That's why athletes load up on carbs before a competition, to supply their muscles with fuel. Processed carbs, on the other hand, that are found in white breads, pasta and cakes, white rice and refined sugar and other processed foods lack the nutrient density found in whole carbs.

GOOD Complex Carbs	BAD Simple Carbs
High in fiber	Low in fiber/nutrients
Metabolism booster	Empty cals turn to fat
Feel fuller, longer	Feel tired
Food Examples	**Food Examples**
Whole grain bread	White bread
Brown rice	Sugar, brown/white
Quinoa	Fruit juices
Fruits	White rice
Sweet potato	Pretzels/chips
Vegetables	Sugary cereals

In his best-selling book, **The Starch Solution**, Dr. John McDougall writes about some of the benefits of consuming complex (good) carbohydrates:

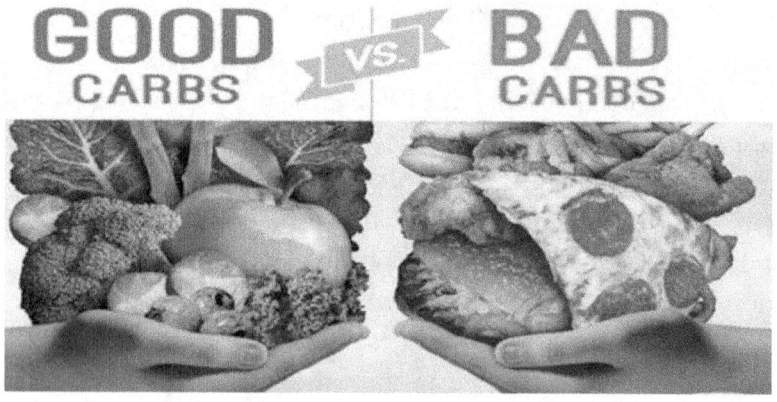

"Carbohydrates help us to radiate vitality. Every year millions of people lose weight without necessarily improving their health. In fact, these weight-loss methods often cause illness. These diets work by severe carbohydrate deprivation, which causes a state of illness and when people become sick they lose their appetite and lose weight. This method of losing weight is analogous to the weight loss seen in people taking cancer chemotherapy drugs.

A carbohydrate based diet, on the other hand, brings radiant health along with the loss of excess body fat. Endurance athletes know the benefits

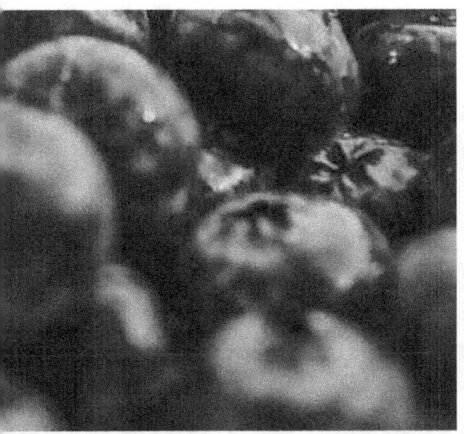

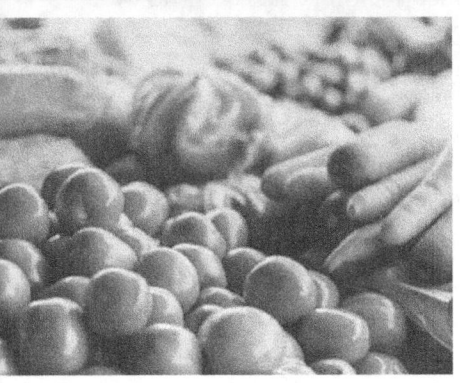

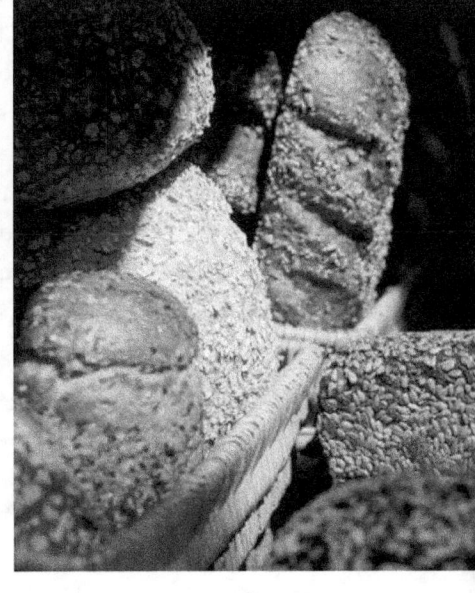

of "carbo loading." In addition to enabling peak performance, a carbohydrate based diet improves blood flow to all tissues in the body. The skin glows with a clear complexion from the improved circulation. A welcome by-product is the elimination of oily skin, blackheads, whiteheads and acne. From weight loss and the resulting relief from arthritis, people on a carbohydrate based diet feel active, agile, and more youthful."

DIABETES 2: IT'S NOT THE SUGAR... IT'S THE FAT!
PART 1

When I see so much conflicting and often confusing information on nutrition, I feel very privileged to be experiencing and discovering how important a role nutrition has in preventing and reversing certain chronic diseases...caused by the Standard American Diet. The main problem, as I have expressed in recent posts, is not that doctors don't recognize the importance of eating healthy, the problem is that they don't understand how significant a role nutrition actually plays. To a great extent, this is because of lack of personal experience as well as the decision to not further their education once the diploma is on the wall.

Case in point – TYPE 2 DIABETES

The 2010 Banting Memorial Lecture was delivered by Professor D.R. Mathews to the Annual Professional Conference of Diabetes UK, Liverpool, on March 4, 2010.

He states:

"We are currently facing a global pandemic of obesity and Type 2 diabetes. In some settings, the population prevalence of Type 2 diabetes is 50%, and half of those affected will die from diabetes-related complications. Eight centuries ago, an epidemic of bubonic plague swept across Europe,

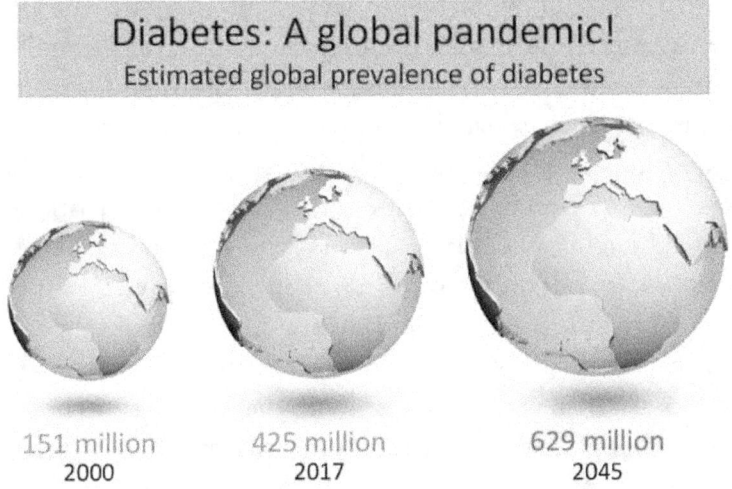

Diabetes: A global pandemic!
Estimated global prevalence of diabetes

| 151 million | 425 million | 629 million |
| 2000 | 2017 | 2045 |

International Diabetes Federation. IDF Diabetes Atlas. 8ᵗʰ Edition. 2017

killing at least half of its victims. We here draw comparisons between these two pandemics, proposing close analogies between the 'Black Death' of the 14th century and the modern – day equivalent of Type 2 diabetes."

Most researchers and doctors today acknowledge that diabetes 2 is a pandemic (worldwide epidemic). In the U.S. it has moved up to 3rd place on the list of killer diseases (Boston University, University of Pennsylvania, 2017) while in Mexico it's now number one (Global Burden of Disease Project, 2017). Interestingly the US and Mexico also rank 1 and 2 in obesity. The predictions are that diabetes 2 will be the #1 killer globally, within the next few years. Although the disease was previously called adult onset diabetes, it was changed to type 2 diabetes because of the growing number of children being affected.

I'm amazed how many people I've met recently who have the disease or have the precursor, pre-diabetes. Recently, I met a woman at a friend's house who had the disease and was told by her doctor that she will be on medication for the rest of her life, included insulin. I began to talk to her about the personal experiences of many doctors and health practitioners who are having undeniable success with diet and diabetes 2. **Patients are not only surviving...they are thriving!** I spoke to her about the real cause of the disease, which is not the same explanation given by most doctors... that sugar overload in the bloodstream is the problem. With that conclusion, the goal is to keep sugar levels under control with drugs...often including the use of insulin.

Patients are told that diabetes 2 is progressive and the ultimate goal is to control the symptoms as best as possible. As a result, doctors keep their patients on drugs for the remainder of their shortened lives, lives that are filled with the potential dangers of leg amputations, blindness, kidney failure, alzheimers and heart and other chronic diseases.

What is the alternative?

According to the "wise" doctors, the first step is to recognize that the problem with the disease is not the increase of sugar in the bloodstream...that's merely a symptom. The real problem is the buildup of fat, primarily in the muscles and liver, that blocks the sugar from entering the cells in order to provide the energy needed for normal functioning. If the sugar can't enter the cells, via the insulin, produced by the pancreas, then it remains in the blood. This leads to insulin resistance, where the insulin is no longer able to perform its role.

If this situation continues…blood sugar levels rise and need to be controlled. If the cause of the problem, as I mentioned, is the excess fat covering the muscles, which blocks the sugar from entering and providing energy, and not the sugar in the blood itself, then it seems to make sense that, if we eliminate the fat, we can open the door to our muscle cells, so that the sugar can enter and do its job. Once normal sugar levels return, diabetes 2 can, in most cases, be completely reversed. This may sound so extraordinarily simple that we may eventually need a book titled *"Reversing Type 2 Diabetes for Dummies."*

In Part 2, I'll discuss further the key for reversing Type 2 Diabetes

DIABETES 2: IT'S NOT THE SUGAR… IT'S THE FAT!
PART 2

If I were to ask you the question, "What do you want?", what would be your response? You could say, "I want more money or a new house or a new car or a new wife or husband, etc.?"

But, if I ask you, "what do you *really* want?", then you would probably mull over the question a little bit more… trying to touch a deeper meaning inside. Finally, your response could be more like, "I want to be happy" or, "I want to be in peace and harmony" or, "I just want to feel good." Because, if you're not feeling well, on a deeper level, then how much can you really enjoy all those other things you said you wanted? That brings us to a hypothetical question, "what does your body want?" Could it be fundamentally the same as what you want… to be happy, to be in peace and harmony, to feel good? The very fact that our physical body and it's immune system is constantly fighting to be comfortable and to be free of disease and pain, seems to support that train of thought.

Just as we need to be reminded of what we *really* want, we also need to be reminded of what our body really wants, beyond the taste of the food we put in our mouths…and that is to be healthy. The body's desire to be healthy is so powerful that, not only does it make unceasing efforts to avoid illness and disease, but also strives to reverse any diseases we may already have. And this can happen if we help it by not getting in it's way. As a result, little by little, we can improve our relationship with our body. We can listen to it and respond to it's needs and, in turn, we will receive the gift of good health. And it's not only the chronic diseases that we can protected from but also the protection against and quick recovery from the colds and flus that bother us every year.

Reversing type 2 diabetes

Because it is now becoming a pandemic and has had such a devastating effect on children worldwide, the reversal of this disease needs to become a medical priority. Wouldn't it be wonderful if our doctor told us that we have two options with regards to our diabetes 2. 1) We can continue to take the prescribed medicines for the rest of our lives with the hope of not succumbing to the painful ravages of the disease or 2) we change our eating habits and have a very good chance to be free of the disease, within a short period of time. Although, unfortunately, most doctors will not give us the options, there are those that will. They are the ones who carry the hope as well as the experience of reversing the disease.

Dr. John McDougall:

"Drug therapy has consistently failed patients with type-2 diabetes, and their well- intended doctors, making the search for an alternative treatment imperative. Since the rich Western diet is agreed to be the cause of this epidemic, should diet not be the first place to look for the prevention and the cure? Written reports on the benefits of a low- fat, high-carbohydrate, plant-food-based diet on type-2 diabetes date back to at least 1930. Several published studies demonstrate how type-2 diabetics can stop insulin and get off diabetic oral medications with a change in diet. One goalpost is weight loss to the point of normal body weight, at this time the blood sugars of most patients diagnosed with type-2 diabetes will become normal, and then everyone will agree that no further treatment with medications is needed.

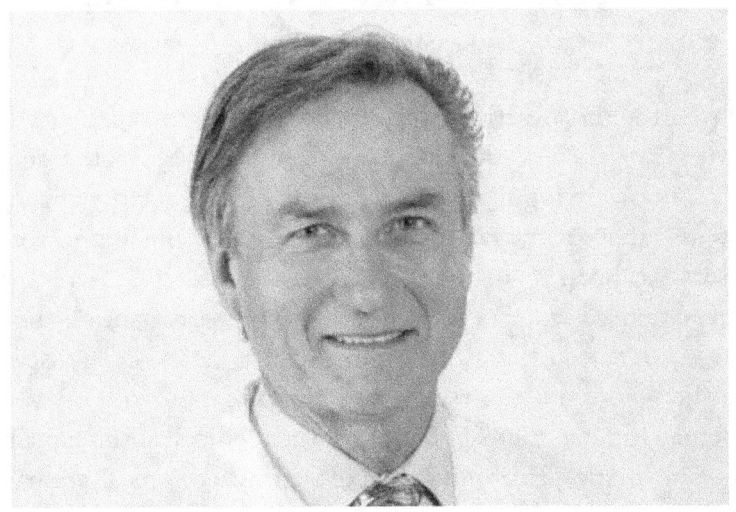

Dr. John McDougall

By great good fortune, this same low-fat, no-cholesterol diet success-fully used for diet-therapy for diabetes has been shown to prevent and treat heart and kidney disease, and prevent many common forms of cancer. Heart disease accounts for 70% of the deaths in diabetics, diabetes is the number one cause of kidney failure, and cancer is more common in diabetics.

Uninformed and purposely misled, as is the case now, the patient cannot get well and the doctor is ineffective in carrying out his or her duties. Consideration for the truth, and the appropriate medical practices that must follow, would change the entire healthcare system for the good, reducing costs and improving patient outcomes substantially."

In Part 3, you'll read about what other "wise" doctors have to say about reversing Type 2 Diabetes.

DIABETES 2: IT'S NOT THE SUGAR...
IT'S THE FAT!
PART 3

Maybe the most difficult concept for people to accept is that reversal of chronic diseases is not only possible but is actually a re-occurring fact. This is especially true for the chronic diseases that are most effected by what we eat, including heart disease, cancer, high blood pressure and diabetes 2. Yes, we can sometimes control diseases and in some cases, bring about remission for short periods of time, but to claim that a disease can be reversed is not something that will easily roll off your doctor's tongue. It's just not part of the medical culture and it's not information that one would expect to see or hear about... in the media.

For Diabetes 2 – Part 3, the following are some comments from...

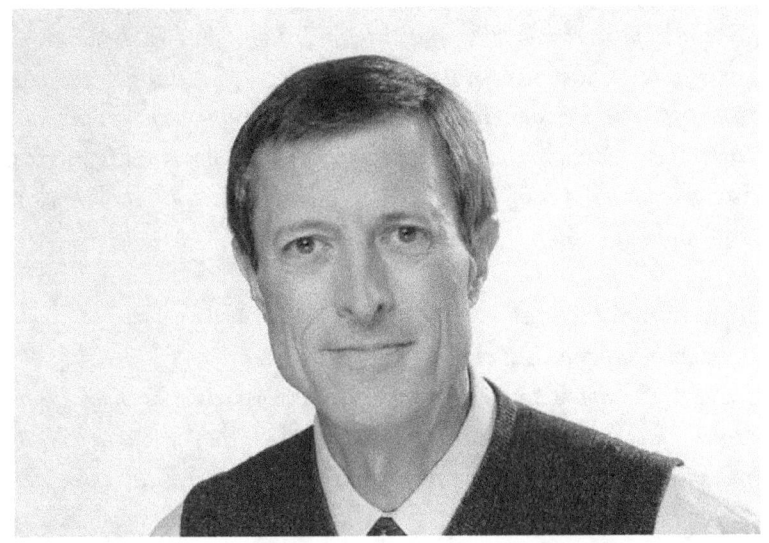

Dr. Neal Bernard

Dr. Neal Bernard –

http://www.pcrm.org

"Blood sugar levels are high in diabetes, so a common idea has held that eating sugar somehow triggers the disease process. However, the major diabetes organizations take a different view. The American Diabetes Association1 and Diabetes UK2 have labelled this notion a "myth," as has the Joslin Diabetes Center,3 which wrote, "Diabetes is not caused by eating too much sugar." These and other organizations have worked to educate people about the causes of diabetes and the role that foods play in the disease process.

Type 2 diabetes typically starts with insulin resistance. That is, the cells of the body resist insulin's efforts to escort glucose into the cells. What causes insulin resistance? It appears to be caused by an accumulation of microscopic fat particles within muscle and liver cells.4 This fat comes mainly from the diet—chicken fat, beef fat, cheese fat, fish fat, and even vegetable fat. To try to overcome insulin resistance, the pancreas produces extra insulin. When the pancreas can no longer keep up, blood sugar rises. The combination of insulin resistance and pancreatic cell failure leads to type 2 diabetes."

Dr. Michael Greger –
http://www.nutritionfacts.org

"Type 2 diabetes has been referred to as the 21st century's Black Death in terms of its exponential spread around the world and devastating health impacts. Instead of the bubonic plague, though, its pathological agents may be high-fat and high-calorie diets. Type 2 diabetes, however, is almost always preventable, often treatable, and sometimes even reversible through diet and lifestyle changes. Like other leading killers—especially heart disease and high blood pressure—type 2 diabetes may be an unfortunate consequence of dietary choices. There is hope, though, even if you already have diabetes. Through lifestyle changes, you may be able to achieve a complete remission of type 2 diabetes, even if you've been suffering with the disease for decades.

People who eat a plant-based diet have been found to have just a small fraction of the diabetes rate seen in those who regularly eat meat. As diets become increasingly plant-based, there appears to be a stepwise drop in diabetes rates. Based on a study of 89,000 Californians, flexitarians (who eat meat maybe once weekly rather than daily) appear to cut their rate of diabetes by 28 percent, and those who cut out all meat except fish appear to cut their rates in half. What about those eliminating all meat, including fish? They appear to eliminate 61 percent of their risk. And those who go a step farther and drop eggs and dairy, too? They may drop their diabetes rates 78 percent compared with people who eat meat on a daily basis."

T. Colin Campbell, Phd –
http://www.nutritionstudies.org

"*Modern drugs and surgery offer no cure for diabetics. At best, current drugs allow diabetics to maintain a reasonably functional lifestyle, but these drugs will never treat the cause of the disease. As a consequence, diabetics face a lifetime of drugs and medications, making diabetes an enormously costly disease. The economic toll of diabetes in the U.S.: over $245 billion in 2013, up from $113 billion in 2000.*

But there is hope. In fact there is much more than hope, if we simply keep an open mind. The food we eat has enormous influence over this disease. The right diet not only prevents but also treats diabetes. What then is the "right" diet? All findings support the idea that both across and within populations, high fiber, whole plant based foods protect against diabetes, and high fat, high protein, animal based foods promote diabetes."

In this life we need to be properly educated, which means to be fully informed. If not, then the possibility of making the right choices, becomes extremely limited. With regards to health education and nutrition, if we do not have enough right information, how can we make intelligent and conscious choices? I hope that this 3 part series, including the input from the "wise" doctors, has shed enough light on the topic of type 2 diabetes, that it becomes an eye opener for those suffering with the disease as well as for the general public.

HOW HEALTHY ARE OILS?
PART 1

The other day I was in the supermarket and while meandering through the aisles I was really impressed by the amount and variety of different oils being offered to us...the consumer.

When I see so much of any particular food along those aisles, I see the stamp of multi-billion dollar businesses as well as major consumer purchasing. The questions I ask myself is, how healthy is oil...anyways?

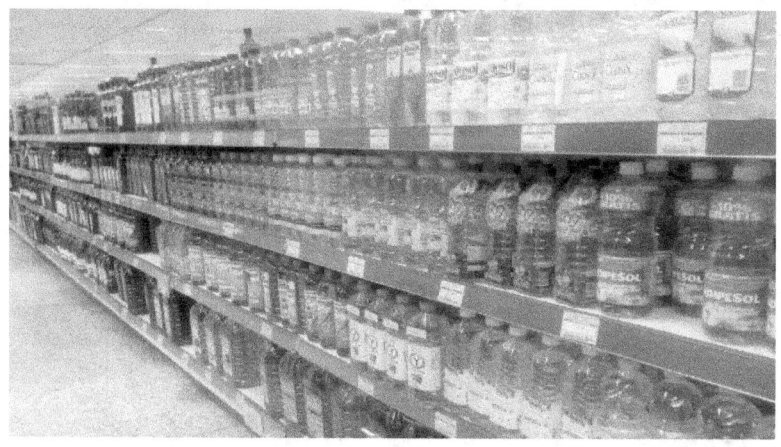

As is the case with processed sugar, all oils are heavily processed and as a result lose almost all of their nutrients that were available in the original fruit, nut or seed. These include vitamins, minerals, fiber, proteins and anti-oxidants. What we're left with is mostly 100% liquid fat. With 120 calories per tablespoon, oils are one of the most fattening, calorically dense foods on the planet. Just put 3 tablespoons on your tossed salad and you've reached 20% of the recommended calorie intake for the day.

But the story doesn't end there.

The endothelium, which is the inner lining of our blood vessels, secretes nitric oxide, a substance that promotes the flexibility that the vessels need, in order to adapt to the ebb and flow of the blood as it circulates through our bodies. Recent evidence is showing that processed oils damage this one cell thick lining. The result is that production of the nitric oxide decreases while the danger of hardening of the arteries (atherosclerosis), increases. This doesn't only affect the heart but the brain as well, which requires a constant flow of oxygen... to avoid deterioration.

OLIVE OIL:

The olive oil craze began during the 1980s as a result of studies showing that, in general, Europeans were suffering and dying less than Americans from chronic diseases. They were following the "Mediterranean Diet" (MD) which was heathier than the Standard American Diet (SAD). Their diet included more fruits, vegetables and grains than the SAD, which includes more meat, dairy and processed foods. The Europeans also used and still use olive oil. For some reason, for those on the SAD, what was adopted was the olive oil instead of the more nutritious plant based foods. As a result, the health of people on the SAD has continued to degenerate for the past 25 years. Still, olive oil is considered healthy, even among most health professionals.

According to Dr. Caldwell Esselstyn, author of the perennial best seller "Prevent and Reverse Heart Disease", the book behind Bill Clinton's Life – Changing Plant Based Diet:

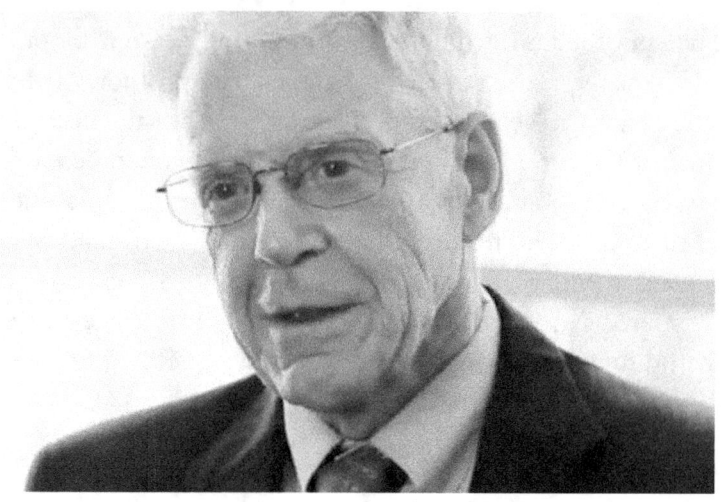

Dr. Caldwell Esselstyn

"No oil! Not even olive oil, which goes against a lot of other advice out there about so called good fats. The reality is that oils are extremely low in nutritive value. Both the mono-unsaturated and saturated fat contained in oils is harmful to the endothelium, the innermost lining of the artery, and that injury is the gateway to vascular disease. It doesn't matter whether it's olive oil, corn oil, coconut oil, canola oil, or any other kind. Avoid ALL oil."

COCONUT OIL

Coconut oil, with its sweet smell of the tropics and its purported claims to cure what ails you, is everywhere. People are using it in their shampoos, skin creams, cooking, and even in their smoothies and coffee. There are even claims that it helps to prevent and cure dementia and alzheimer's. Recent studies are showing the opposite, that these diseases result, at least in part, from vascular problems, stemming from the build up of plaque in the blood vessels to the brain…similar to the relationship between atherosclerosis and heart disease.

A new science advisory in 2017, from the **American Heart Association** recommended against ingesting coconut oil. Frank Sacks, M.D., lead author of the advisory is a professor of cardiovascular disease prevention in the department of nutrition at the Harvard School of Public Health.

The advisory, an analysis of more than 100 published research studies dating as far back as the 1950s, reaffirmed that saturated fats raise LDL, or "bad" cholesterol. Tropical vegetable oils such as coconut oil contain high levels of saturated fats, and the authors reported that coconut oil raised LDL cholesterol in seven controlled trials.

"One of the real problems in transmitting health information is that generally people who are writing about it don't look into what's come before," he said. The media also don't pay much attention to new studies that support or extend current dietary recommendations. "The overall effect has misled the public on the science of dietary fats," he said.

People are also quick to believe trends that aren't supported by science, he said. A prime example is coconut oil, widely touted for its health benefits. "I just don't know" who is pushing it, but it's not scientists, Sacks said. It may be driven by manufacturers looking to profit, or some countries' economic dependence on coconut oil, he said.

According to the advisory, **coconut oil** is 82 percent saturated fat, and studies show it raises LDL "bad" cholesterol as much as butter, beef fat or palm oil.

In "HOW HEALTHY ARE OILS? – Part 2, You will find healthy alternatives to cooking with oil as well as tasty options for salad dressings.

HOW HEALTHY ARE OILS?
PART 2

Cooking without oil is really simple and after 7 years of experiencing my wife Delia's wonderful cooking, I can truly say that you don't need the added taste of oil to make foods taste great. On the contrary, as my taste buds started adapting to the new oil less flavor of each individual vegetable, I actually began to enjoy eating more.

COOKING:

In Delia's own words…

It may seem impossible but it's true: We don't need oil to cook. After seven years of eliminating all fats in the preparation of meals I can truly say that yes, it's possible and very easy to use substitutes for all the oils that we're accustomed to using when cooking our favorite dishes.

Instead of frying, I sauté onions and garlic in the preparation of rice and different sauces, stews or casseroles. I only need to add a little water, wine or vegetable broth and cook over a low flame in a covered pan or pot. It's important to mix the ingredients, once in a while, to prevent the food from sticking. I prefer to use non-stick pots and pans (without the chemical Perfluorooctanoic acid – PFOA), that make it simpler to cook without oil or fat.

For baking successfully without oil you can use mashed bananas or avocado, soaked prunes and even canned pumpkin. Either one will provide the moistness you desire.

To prepare Mexican style dishes, it's not necessary to fry the tortillas, potatoes or other foods. In most cases you can get great and very tasty results grilling instead of frying. Another benefit of cooking without oil is during the cleanup. It's less of a hassle to wash the dishes and pots and pans.

Salad dressing:

It's important to be reminded of something we already know… that with regards to making salads, each vegetable or fruit that we include has it's own unique flavor and that it's a wonderful experience to savor the individual tastes as they explode in our mouths. For that reason I try to make the dressings simple and let the individual vegetables speak for themselves.

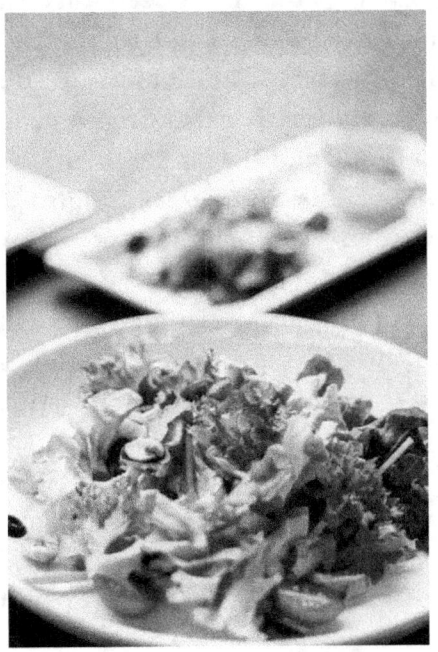

For salad dressing, without added oils, there are so many options available on the internet that one can try a different dressing every day of the week. For me, I keep it simple by alternating between the following 3 options and add different herbs and spices to alternate tastes. In my salads, I'll often include at least 5 of the following ingredients: green leafy vegetables, avocados, beans, tomatoes, onions, carrots, cucumbers, sweet peppers, apple slices, nuts and seeds, dried and unsweetened cranberries.

1) After chopping up the salad ingredients in a bowl, I'll mix in the juice of half a lemon, a tablespoon of natural organic soy sauce (since there's a lot of unhealthy soy sauces out there, please read the labels for additives and coloring), powdered garlic and Italian herb seasoning to taste, a teaspoon of chia seeds and balsamic vinegar. I would then add a few nuts and/or seeds (almond, cashews, macadamia, walnuts, sesame, squash or sunflower seeds).

2) After chopping up the salad ingredients in a bowl, mix in the juice of half a lemon, a tablespoon of natural organic soy sauce, a tablespoon of ground flax seeds, a tablespoon of organic mustard and a teaspoon of agave syrup. Add nuts and/or seeds.

3) To vary I'll often make a salad plate which would include choices from the list of ingredients above. To the salad I would squeeze a half lemon and

sprinkle powdered garlic, herb seasoning, ground flax seeds and a tablespoon of balsamic vinegar.

An added note and for your information:

Like most people, for so many years, before I changed to a whole food vegan diet, I relied on what the supermarket offered and still offers in the form of salad dressings (i.e., Italian, ranch, French, blue cheese, etc.). Just look at the ingredients on the label of one of the most popular brands of Italian dressings:

INGREDIENTS: VINEGAR, VEGETABLE OIL (SOYBEAN AND/OR CANOLA), WATER, SUGAR, SALT, CONTAINS LESS THAN 2% OF GARLIC,* GARLIC, RED BELL PEPPER,* ONION,* ONION, SPICE, XANTHAN GUM, MONOSODIUM GLUTAMATE, NATURAL FLAVOR, LEMON JUICE CONCENTRATE, CALCIUM DISODIUM EDTA (TO PROTECT FLAVOR), ANNATTO EXTRACT (COLOR).

Ingredients are always listed in the order of quantity so you can see that 3 of the first five main ingredients are oil, sugar and salt. The amount of salt per portion in this dressing is already over the daily suggested maximum. According to cravings experts, the combination of fat, sugar and salt are what keeps us addicted to processed foods. That's what keeps us coming back for our fix at McDonalds, Burger King and Pizza Hut. Xanthan gum is used as a thickening agent. Monosodium Glutamate (MSG) is to add flavoring, EDTA is a preservative and Annato extract is used as a coloring agent. It's also used to make medicines to treat diabetes, diarrhea, heartburn, malaria, hepatitis and as a bowel cleanser. Most of the added ingredients are to preserve foods on the shelves...since the product is no longer fresh.

Fortunately, when you make your own salad dressing, you can choose from fresh ingredients, so that you don't need to add chemicals or preservatives.

As a final thought here, I highly suggest acquiring the habit of checking the ingredients on the labels of all processed foods. Be aware of added oils, sugar, salt, preservatives, words that you don't understand and words that begin with the letters "die."

TO SUPPLEMENT OR NOT TO SUPPLEMENT
PART 1

Supplementing with vitamins has to be one of the most controversial nutrition topics. About 10 years ago I became an avid fan of consuming supplements, up to 13 capsules a day, including a multi-vitamin, vitamins A, B complex, C, D and E. It was through a reputable company based in the United States. Living in Mexico I would travel twice a year to load up on their products. I also subscribed to their monthly magazine which was of high quality and included very interesting articles on nutrition and health. About five years ago I became aware of something while reading a couple of the articles. That, although vitamins and minerals were emphasized as the means to prevent and reverse certain illnesses and diseases, foods that contain the specific vitamin or mineral were almost never mentioned as an option. Then, 2 or 3 pages later, I would see an add that would promote the vitamin or mineral supplement that corresponded to the article I had just read. Not only did I see this as a clever way for the business to promote their product but, as a whole food plant based advocate, I asked myself two questions: 1) If whole food plant based nutrition is supposed to provide all the vitamins I need to be in good health, why am I taking so many supplements? And 2) How healthy are supplements, anyway?

Dr. T. Colin Campbell is a world renowned biochemist and author of the NY Times Best Seller **"The China Study"**, which has sold over 2 million copies. The book is considered to be one the most comprehensive studies of nutrition ever conducted. His follow-up book **"Whole, Rethinking the Science of Nutrition"**, explains why, with all the overwhelming evidence showing that a whole food plant based diet is the healthiest human diet, that evidence is not being made readily available to the public? Why are so many people still confused about what to eat?

Dr. Campbell uses the term "Reductionism" to explain the core of the problem with Western Medicine. As a reductionist you believe that everything can be understood if you understand it's component parts. A wholist believes that the whole is greater than the sum of it's parts. An example of this, is the famous Indian fable of the blind men explaining what an elephant is by feeling a particular part. In reality, you can only understand what an elephant is when you see the "whole" elephant.

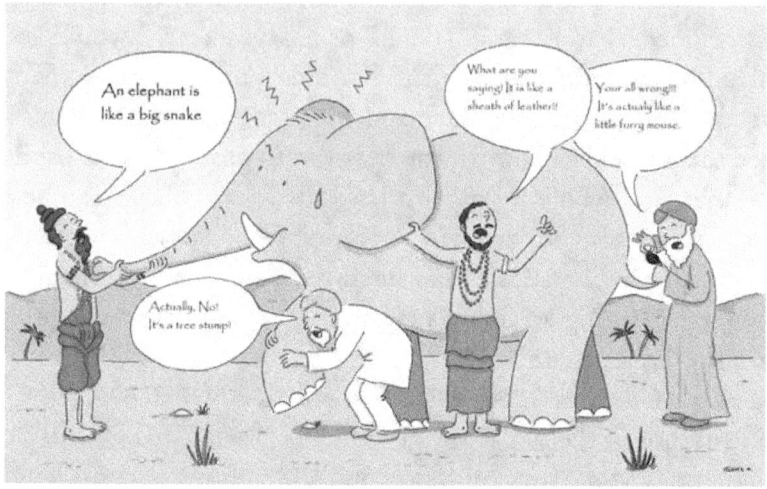

PHARMACEUTICAL DRUGS AND REDUCTIONISM

Before the advent of pharmaceutical drugs, whole plants were used to cure diseases. I remember living with a group of friends in the small village of Xcalak, on the Mexican Caribbean. It was 1967 and one of the group came down with malaria. There were no doctors in the village and since it was a good eight hour sailboat ride to the State capital, Chetumal, the villagers often had to depend on the curative property of the local plants and herbs that grew there. So, we took our friend to the woman who was trained in this herbal knowledge and she prepared a tea from one of the native plants. The result: In 9 days the malaria was gone.

Why am I telling you this?

Well, as scientists began to study the curative power of plants, it occurred to them that maybe they could extrapolate the specific ingredient in the plant that cured the ailment...and reproduce it chemically, in the laboratory. This is a form of reductionism... believing that the specific ingredient was equivalent to the "whole" plant. What's the difference? Well, when our friend drank the tea, during those 9 days, there were no side effects. Today, with chemically produced medicines, it's hard to find one without side effects...some very serious and even fatal.

SUPPLEMENTS AND REDUCTIONISM
Note: I would like to make it clear that I'm referring to vitamin and mineral supplements, not certain herbal supplements (i.e., ginger, turmeric, curcumin, etc.).

Homo sapiens, over their millions of years of existence, have always eaten whole foods. Then, during the 1980s, the supplement industry emerged. The goal, just like with the pharmaceutical industry was to prove that individual vitamins and minerals was the equivalent to the vitamins and minerals in the whole food. In other words, a vitamin C supplement would be equivalent to the vitamin C in a whole apple. Is that true?

According to Dr. Campbell,

"The natural health community has also fallen prey to the ideology that chemicals ripped from their natural context are as good or better than whole foods. Instead of synthesizing the presumed "active ingredients" from medicinal herbs, as done for prescription drugs (often with warnings of life threatening side effects), supplement manufacturers seek to extract and bottle the active ingredients from foods known or believed to promote good health and healing. And just like prescription drugs,

the active agents function imperfectly, incompletely and unpredictably, when divorced from the whole plant food from which they're derived or synthesized. The process of nutrition is profoundly wholistic, in that the way a body uses a particular nutrient depends on what other nutrients are ingested along with it. If we just take an isolated vitamin C pill, we miss out on the cast of "supporting characters" that may give vitamin C it's potency. Even if we add many of these characters into the pill too, which some manufacturers have done with bioflavonoids, we are still assuming that whatever is in the apple and not in the pill is somehow not important."

One of the problems of depending on supplements to provide us with the nutrition we need is that we can believe that we're "off the hook", with regards to eating the right foods. As long as we take our "magic" pill, we can binge on hot dogs, French fries and ice cream.

TO SUPPLEMENT OR NOT TO SUPPLEMENT
PART 2

Just like with pharmaceutical drugs, supplements are a multibillion dollar industry, growing exponentially every decade, since the 1980s. The business has gotten so big that most of the commercial supplements are now produced by big pharma. One of the problems though is that while pharmaceutical drugs are regulated by the FDA, since the Dietary Supplement Health and Education Act, or DSHEA, in 1994, there has been very little regulation of the supplement industry.

"Increasingly, Big Pharma and Big Nutrition are indistinguishable," claims Lynn Stuart Parramore (writer for Salon online magazine). **"The very same mega-companies with**

gigantic chemical labs that make drugs are cooking up vitamin and herbal supplements labeled with sunny terms like 'natural' and 'wholesome.' Pfizer, Unilever, Novartis, GlaxoSmithKline and other big pharmaceutical firms make or sell supplements." While she does acknowledge there are a few small companies still in the mix, Parramore says they represent a tiny amount of the total sales in the $23 billion-a-year supplement business. Many of these pharma companies have made the foray into supplements because it plays to their strengths while being far, far cheaper than drug development.

So how safe are supplements?

In February of 2015, the attorney general of the State of New York investigated and found that top brands of herbal supplements at GNC, Target, Walgreens, and Walmart were fraudulently labelled: the FDA found many pills that did not contain the main active ingredients they claimed on the label. How did this happen? The short answer is that no one checked; and many people were successfully scammed. The unfortunate fact is that supplements (vitamins, minerals, protein powders and herbal extracts) lack the regulation that is provided to both food and medicine.

Before 1994 there were more standards that the supplement companies had to meet. However, the Industry's lobbying and advertising was very successful. People petitioned the Congress and the industry lobbied until the Dietary Supplement Health and Education Act, or DSHEA, was passed. This act prevents the FDA from regulating supplements or their labels.

It actually weakened previous regulatory ability and now the FDA can't act unless they can show a supplement is unsafe; and the burden of proof is on the FDA!

So, if you're thinking about or currently using a dietary supplement, here are some points to keep in mind.
Be aware that an herbal supplement may contain dozens of compounds and that all of its ingredients may not be known. Researchers are studying many of these products in an effort to identify what ingredients may be active and understand their effects in the body. Also consider the possibility that what's on the label may not be what's in the bottle. Analyses of dietary supplements sometimes find differences between labeled and actual ingredients.

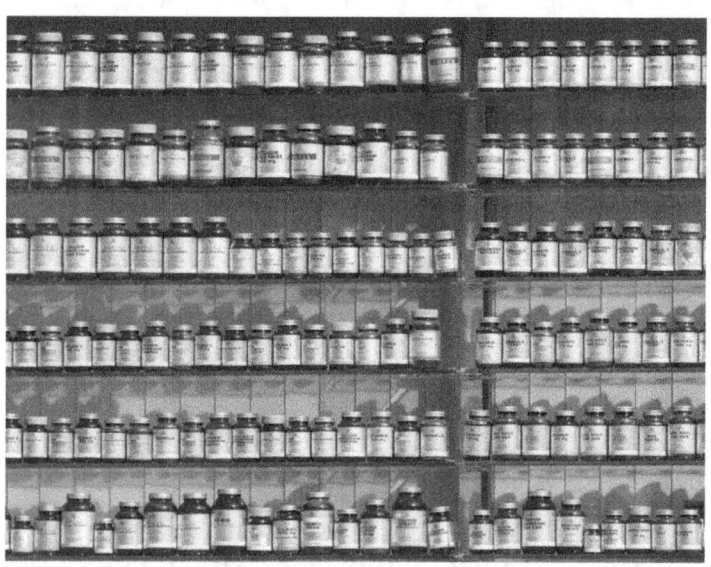

For example:

- An herbal supplement may not contain the correct plant species.
- The amounts of the ingredients may be lower or higher than the label states. That means you may be taking less—or more—of the dietary supplement than you realize.
- The dietary supplement may be contaminated with other herbs, pesticides, or metals, or even adulterated with unlabeled, illegal ingredients such as rescription drugs.

One of the reasons why we take vitamins and minerals is because we believe that foods of today are not as nutrient rich as they were decades ago and that the poor condition of soil these days means that what we eat today is drained of nutrients from years of over farming. Along comes the supplement company to convince us that "no problem"…my supplement will provide you with the missing nutrients.

Is that true?
According to Dr. John McDougall, it's not.

In his acclaimed book, The Starch Solution, he states that *"Plants synthesize vitamins; they are not in the soil. If a plant is going to bear roots, seeds, flowers and/or fruits fit for sale in your market, then it's going to have to produce all of the organic chemicals that is necessary for it's own survival. We call the plant-derived organic chemicals vital for human nutrition vitamins."* And with regards to mineral deficiency, he goes on to say, *"Your risk of suffering from mineral deficiency caused by deleted soil is so incredibly small that a single case would make national headlines. That's because you eat foods grown in a wide variety of soil: corn grown in Nebraska, grapes from Chile, bananas from Panama, and so forth. People take supplements to protect against unfounded fears of developing deficiencies, and false hopes of preventing and curing illnesses that those deficiencies have never been known to cause (for example, heart disease and cancer)."*

TO GLUTEN OR NOT TO GLUTEN

This morning I had breakfast with a good friend of mine at Lolita's restaurant in San Miguel de Allende, Mexico. I told him that I was going to write this post about the non- gluten movement that has taken center stage on the world nutrition platform…so much so that, within the last decade, the non-gluten food industry has blossomed into a $6 billion dollar business. Today, more than 100 million Americans consume gluten-free products. It's estimated that more than half of the people who buy foods labeled gluten-free do not have a clear understanding of what gluten actually is (a protein found in wheat, rye, barley and sometimes in oats), and they consume it because they think it will help them lose weight, because they seem to feel better or because they mistakenly believe they are sensitive to gluten. It can also be found in oats that are grown close to those grains.

As a result, a score of books have been written during the last few years, extolling the incredible benefits from a non-gluten diet. A couple of them (The Grain Brain and Wheat Belly) have become NY Times Best Sellers even though some of the information and research, supporting the authors' conclusions, is now considered highly questionable. After all, the cultivation and harvesting of wheat, which began thousands of years ago, has been sustaining great civilizations since then…

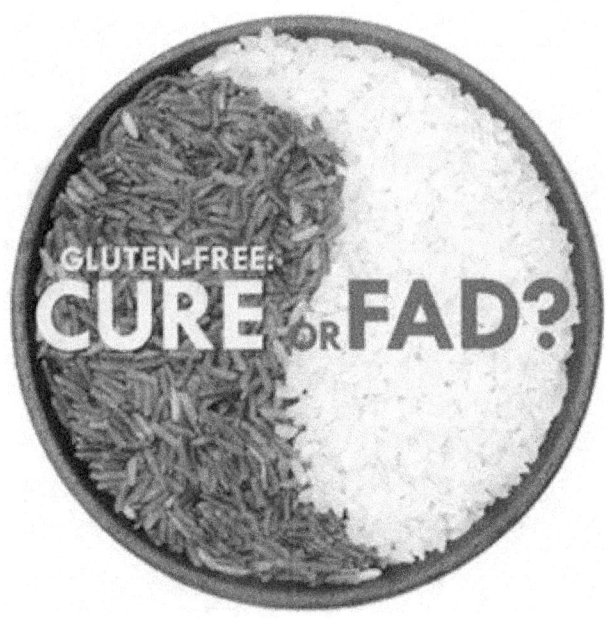

including the ancient Egyptians. So, even with all the hullaba-loo surrounding it, how sure can we be that non-gluten is all what it's cracked up to be?

Getting back to my "breakfast" friend, he commented that his wife has been feeling much better since going gluten free. I responded with, "Is your wife completely sure that she's feeling better because she dropped the gluten or could there be other factors responsible for the improvement"? In other words, maybe people who were previously on the Standard American Diet (SAD) are not feeling better because of the non-gluten foods, but because they're actually eating healthier (i.e., more vegetables, fruits, non-gluten grains and less processed foods).

So, what are the pros and cons of going gluten-free?

PROS:

- Substitution of processed and refined foods with more fruits, vegetables and non-gluten grains…making it healthier than the Standard Western Diet of meat, dairy, eggs and processed and refined foods.
- Avoidance of sugary foods, high fructose corn syrup, sodas and fruit juices.
- Being more selective with our choices of what we eat.
- Paying more attention to the ingredients in the foods we consume.
- Many people feel better on a gluten-free diet.

CONS:

- Research and studies show that only 2% of the population suffers from gluten problems (celiac disease, wheat sensitivity or wheat allergy).
- Since the gluten-free movement is new, it's impossible to know the long term effects of gluten restriction.
- The reason health professionals don't want to see people on gluten-free diets, unless absolutely necessary, is that for the overwhelming majority of people that don't have gluten issues, whole grains—including the gluten grains wheat, barley and rye—are health promoting, linked to the reduced risk of coronary heart disease, cancer, diabetes, obesity and other chronic diseases.
- Proponents of gluten free diets often ban legumes (beans, lentils, chick peas and soy), which are a powerhouse of proteins, nutrients and fiber.

- There is some evidence to suggest that a gluten-free diet may adversely affect gut health in those without celiac disease or gluten sensitivity or allergy. Glutens feed our good bacteria, which may boost immune function and viral infections.
- Gluten withdrawal may undermine the ability to pick up celiac disease, the much more serious form of gluten intolerance. Without consuming gluten celiac disease may not be detected.
- Many so-called gluten-free diets inadvertently still include gluten. Sometimes there's contamination of gluten-free products, so even foods labeled quote-unquote gluten-free may not be.
- There's a lot of non-gluten junk food out there...to be avoided...if you want to be healthy.

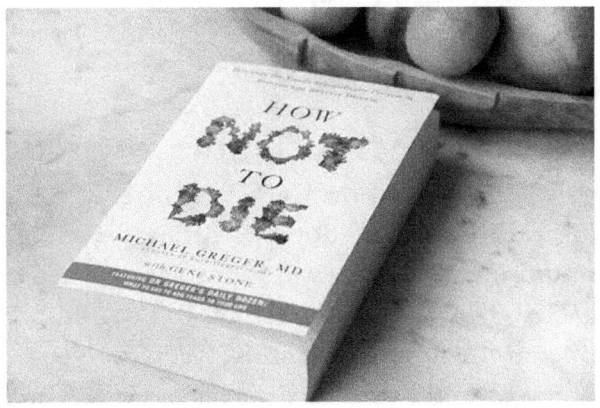

There are 3 legitimate health reasons for eliminating gluten foods from the diet: Celiac Disease, Wheat Sensitivity or Wheat Allergy.

According to Dr. Michael Greger, author of the NY Times best seller *"How Not to Die"*, these problems effect only 2% of the U.S. population. "For the 98% that don't have wheat issues, there is no evidence to suggest that following a gluten-free diet has any benefits."

So what's the best course of action to take if you suspect you might be sensitive to gluten?

Dr. Greger goes on the say: "First off, do not go on a gluten-free diet. If you suffer from chronic irritable bowel type symptoms, such as bloating, abdominal pain and irregular bowel habits, ask your doctor about getting a formal evaluation for celiac disease. If you have celiac, then go on a strict gluten-free diet. If you don't have the disease, the current recommendation is that you first try a healthier diet that includes more fruits, vegetables, whole grains, and beans, all the while avoiding processed foods. The reason people may feel better on a gluten-free diet... and therefore conclude that they may have a problem with gluten... is because they've suddenly stopped eating so much fast food and other processed junk food."

THE PALEO DIET -
Another Low Carb Disguise?

A man is waiting in the doctor's office for a diagnosis. The doctor emerges and says, "I 'm sorry to tell you but you have cancer. The man replies, "I'd like a second opinion" and the doctor responds, "You're ugly too!"

The problem is that opinions are like noses...everyone has one. That's especially the case nowadays with regards to the topic of nutrition on Social Media which is giving us access to a constant flow of enormous amounts of information. There are so many online summits, documentaries, symposiums and websites, on the subject, which seem to attract a lot of attention and viewers. I don't see how providing the opinions of so many so-called experts who all have different opinions would, in any way, help anyone. I used to join these online seminars only to find them confusing because of the conflicting opinions, each in the name of health and well being.

The main problem is that many of these "experts" actually recommend approaches to nutrition that are not necessarily healthful. How can we know if someone is an expert or not? Is it because they're a doctor or wrote a book or have a popular website? After all, if a person is a featured speaker at a conference doesn't that make him or her an expert? Not necessarily. While some people can tell the difference, someone who's new to the topic of diet and nutrition may not be able to. To them all featured speakers would sound like experts. As a result, in so many cases, the only thing that these different opinions create is doubt, confusion, misunderstanding and frustration. In the end people are afraid to make any change at all.

Recently, there was a Doctor's presentation here in San Miguel de Allende, Mexico on the topic of Alzheimers Disease and it's relation to diet. Although I didn't have the opportunity to attend the lecture, I did check out the guest speaker's website, which covered various health topics and their relation to nutrition. Although I was in agreement with some of the Doctor's opinions, there were critical areas where I was not. At the healthy age of 76, the following is my perspective…based on my research and personal experience following a Whole

Food Plant Based diet for the past 8 years, preceded by 32 years as a vegetarian.

On her website the doctor outlines the dos and don'ts of a healthy diet, not only to prevent Alzheimers, but other chronic illnesses as well. On the healthy side, which I wholeheartedly support, she calls for the elimination of processed foods and dairy. What I don't support is her insistence that eating meat (in abundance) is an important component of a healthy diet while consuming whole grains, beans, lentils, chick peas and cruciferous vegetables (i.e., broccoli, cauliflower, Brussel sprouts, kale) are not.

According to her, carbohydrates, refined or not, should be avoided. On her website she shows her complete support for low carbs and even No Carbs. This goes against everything I've personally experienced and researched during these past years. I found that the Doctor's beliefs are very similar to proponents of one the latest diet fads...The Paleo Diet, based on a book that was first published in 2002 and written by Loren Cordain. an exercise physiology professor at Colorado State University. It basically emphasizes a high protein (from animals), saturated fat and low carb diet. It's actually a spinoff of other previous and what I consider "unsustainable" low carb diets...such as Atkins, South Beach, Eat Right for Your Type and Enter the Zone. Why they are unsustainable is because the great majority who go on these diets, mainly to lose weight, last for a few weeks or at best a few months...eventually returning to their original eating habits, which were not very healthy to begin with. Maybe you or someone you know has had this experience. Furthermore, I found a lot of vague and controversial information regarding *1) the benefits of the low carb diet she recommends and 2) the shortcomings of Whole Food Plant Based Nutrition.*

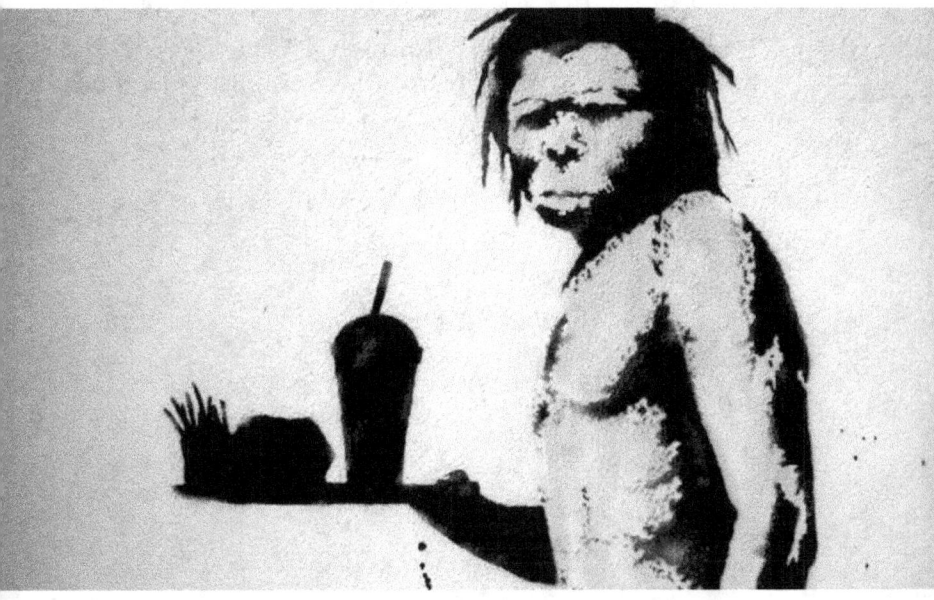

Bansky, "The Caveman"

On her website, the Dr. replies to the question, Do Vegans Live Longer?

"All we have are epidemiological observations to attempt to answer this question, but these do not show any difference in mortality between vegans and omnivores."

First of all, the term "vegan" itself is vague, because eating vegan doesn't mean you're eating healthy. Eating a daily diet of cupcakes, donuts, french fries and refined and processed plant foods is vegan but not much healthier than the Standard American Diet that leads to the chronic diseases that we know so well. Instead, what she needs to consider is a Whole Food Plant Based Diet. With that difference we can say that there definitely are populations in the world that not only live longer but are almost free of the same chronic diseases that cause us so much suffering and premature death. We're talking about the people living in rural China, Japan and Africa as well as the populations discovered by National Geographic's Dan Buettner in the world's Blue Zones:

- The Italian island of Sardinia.
- Okinawa, Japan.
- Loma Linda, California.
- Costa Rica's isolated Nicoya Peninsula.
- Ikaria, an isolated Greek island.

These people all eat a Whole Food Plant Based Diet!!

With Regards to the Paleo Diet:

1) Loren Cordain's conclusions regarding what the Hunter – Gatherers ate during the stone age is based on what present day Hunter- Gatherers eat (70% meat). Previously, in 1968, Richard Lee and anthropologist Richard Daly published an article based on the study of 58 hunter gatherer societies. They found that only 33% of the consumed foods were animal based. Until Codain's findings this was the consensus among

anthropologists. How can we know for sure which is closer to the truth?

2) Since Cordain makes his claims from present day Hunter – Gatherers. Can we be sure that their diet is the same as Paleolithic Man?

3) Because there is doubt as to how long Paleo man lived there is no way we can know if they lived long enough to get chronic diseases. Thus, we really don't know how healthy they actually were as a result of the foods they were consuming.

4) With its focus on consuming large quantities of meat, the new paleo diet could be a poor imitation of the diet of early humans. We've been evolving for 25 million years since our common great ape ancestor, during which time our nutrient requirements and digestive physiology were set down, and therefore probably little affected by our hunter-gatherer days which was at the tail end (2.5 million years). So what were we eating for the first 90% of our evolution? What the great apes ended up eating – over 95% plants.

5) Unfortunately the Paleo dietary pattern also ignores:
   a) the numerous health risks associated with eating meat (high cholesterol and saturated fat, no fiber or antioxidants).
   b) the moral and ethical issues associated with an increased demand for food animals from the Factory Farms.
   c) the effects that eating meat has on the environmental (pollution of the atmosphere from farm

animal gases, pollution of the earth and rivers from farm animal waste, destruction of forests in order to plant grains to feed animals... instead of humans.

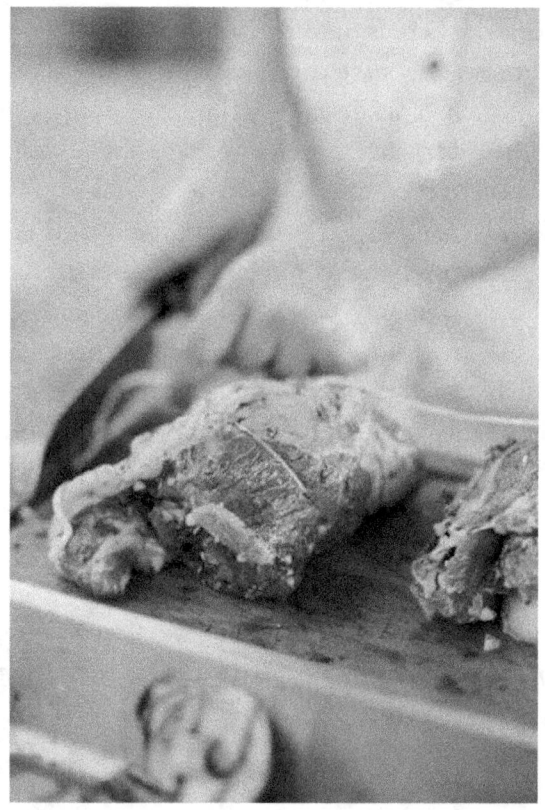

I believe that once we decide on a nutrition path to follow we need to find out if it's right for us...and that is by our experience and personal observation.

What are the results? Am I feeling better? Do I have more energy? Are there certain foods that don't agree with me? These are some of the questions we need to ask ourselves...on our way to the destination of optimal health and wellbeing. In the end...we can become our own experts.

4

DOCTORS, DRUGS AND THE MEDICAL PROFESSION

"It must be frustrating to survive the gauntlet that is our western medical schooling system only to one day come to the realization that you have been taught to only manage illness and disease instead of curing it."

Gary Hopkins, author of "The Master Within"

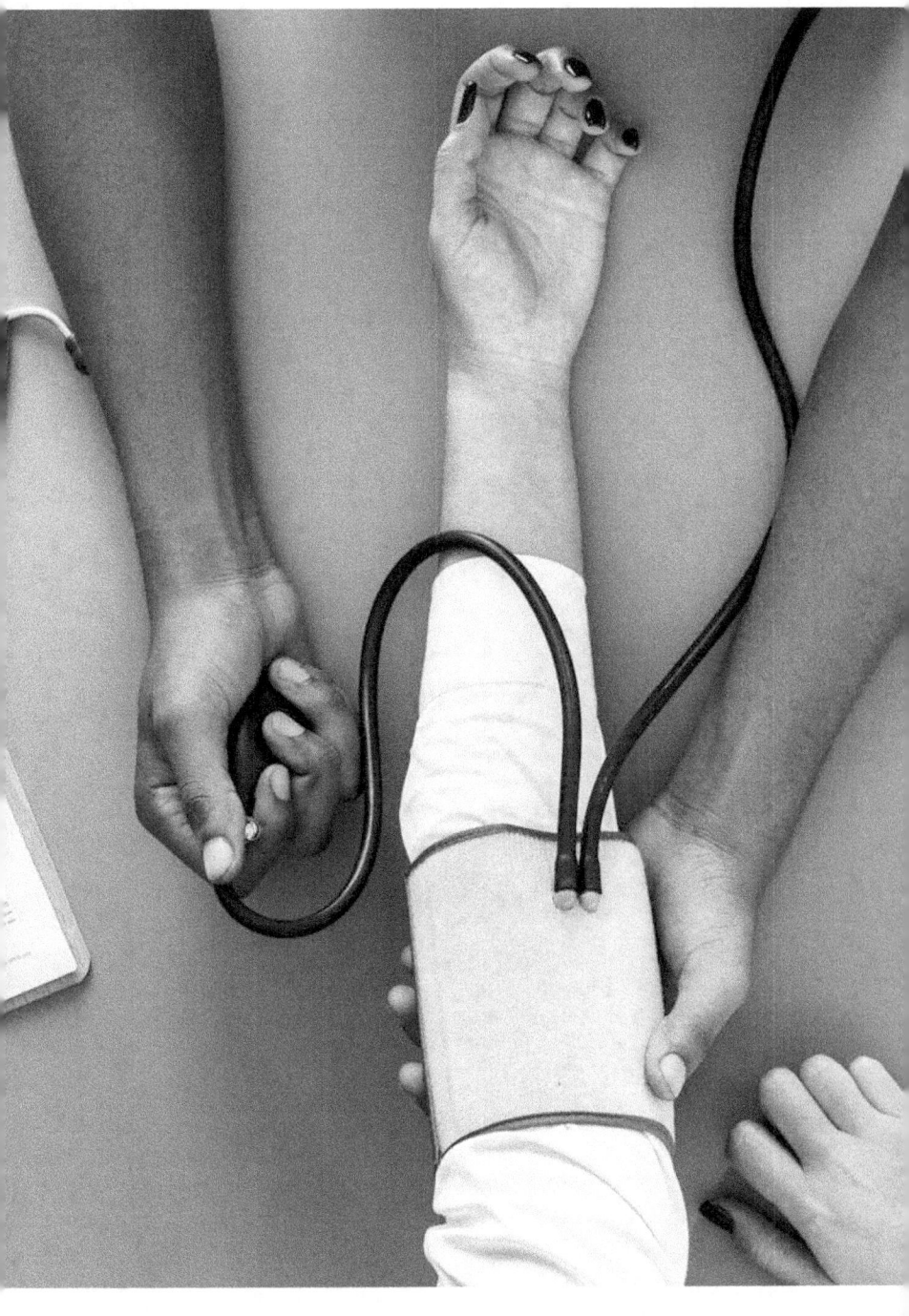

THE THIRD LEADING CAUSE OF DEATH

What most people don't know is that the medical profession, including doctors, drugs and hospitals, is the 3rd leading cause of death in the United States…. producing over 400,000 annual deaths, only exceeded by heart disease and cancer (Journal of the American Medical Association).

Third leading cause of death in U.S.

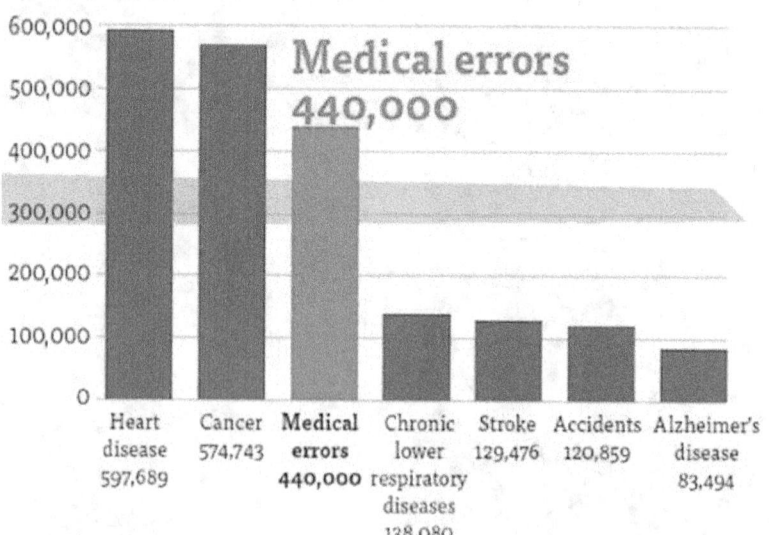

The reasons for this are:

- *Patients not following medication indications*
- *Wrong medications given to patients*
- *Infections acquired in hospitals*
- *Unnecessary surgeries*
- *Errors in surgery*
- *Prescription drug side effects (over 200,000)*

This is well documented information that members of the medical profession are aware of and we are not. Why are we not aware of this data? Is this being kept from us? Well, for one thing, imagine if you had this this information. Might you not look at doctors, hospitals and prescription drugs from a different perspective and with more scrutiny?

Now, don't get me wrong. I never underestimate the important role of doctors. For example, their value is obvious when it comes to:

- Diagnosis
- Repairing fractures
- Healing wounds
- Curing infections with medication
- Relieving pain and discomfort with medication
- Removing the symptoms of illness and chronic disease
- Saving lives through chemotherapy, surgery and radiation

And I said to my body, softly: 'I want to be your friend'. It took a long breath, and replied: 'I have been waiting my whole life for this'.

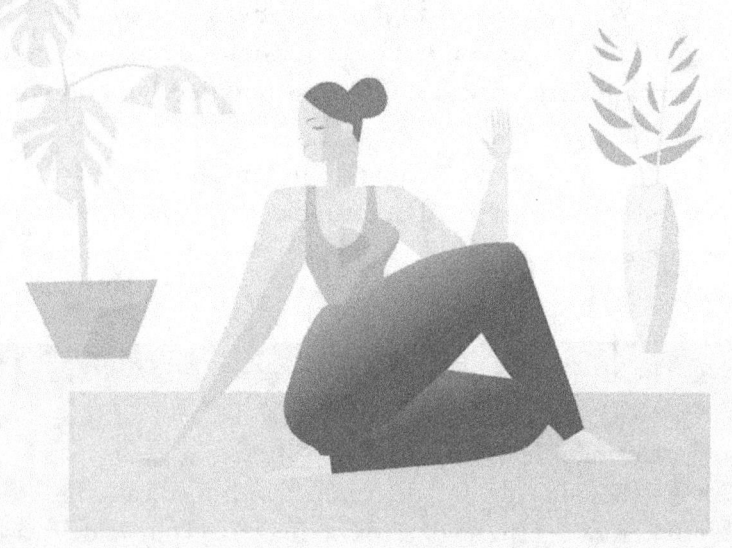

However, when it comes to preventing and even reversing chronic diseases, before they actually happen, the great majority of doctors are not prepared for that, simply because that was not a priority of their education.

So, if that statement is true, what can we do to prevent and reverse diseases? First of all, we need to accept that the solution is mainly up to us...that we're the ones that will make a difference. That we're the ones that need to empower ourselves with the responsibility of doing all we can do, to remain healthy.

It's so important to remember that our body is our friend. It's objective is to be in harmony and when it is, we feel good...with no pain or discomfort. We feel so comfortable that we don't even notice it and we "know" that this physical state is the way it's supposed to be. Yet, to achieve this state of wellbeing our bodies are involved in a constant war (24/7) with external and internal invaders that are trying to dethrone it's protective army...the immune system. The results: Illness and disease, whether it be the flu, the common cold or a more serious threat. So, while we're dealing with our life's circumstances and problem solving, we are oblivious to the battles that our "friend" is constantly involved in...just to keep us healthy.

So, our responsibility actually is to help our body fight it's "battles" by not getting in it's way...and by adopting healthy lifestyle habits such as exercising, avoiding stress and most important...making plant powered foods the foundation of our health. If we do this then we will most probably reduce our dependency on the medical profession to tell us what we need to do and rely more on our own understanding? Think of some of the perks! Less worry and fear about getting sick, feeling healthier and with more energy, reaching one's ideal weight, having the potencial of living a longer, healthier life and spending less money on medical care.

GET TO KNOW YOUR INNER DOCTOR
You know your family doctor, your dentist, your skin doctor, but did you ever meet the doctor within you?

Sound strange?

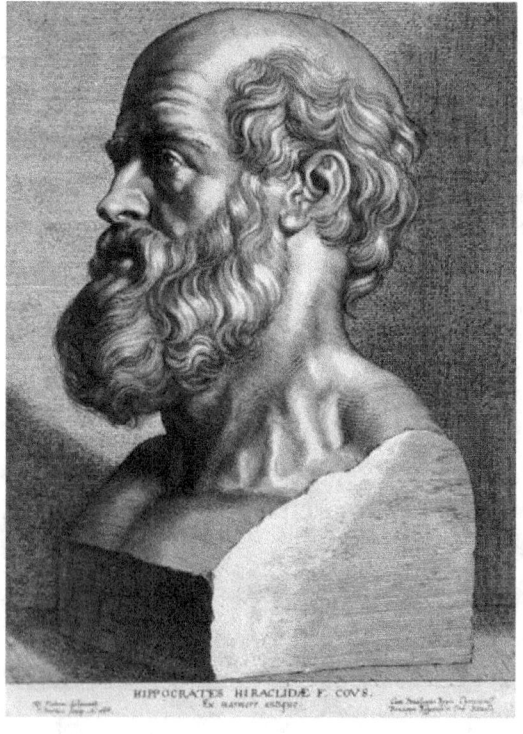

HIPPOCRATES HIRACLIDÆ F. COVS.
Ex antiqvo exemplari

Well, to find out what I'm referring to we need to travel back 2,500 years...to the time of the Greek physician, **Hippocrates**, a doctor who is so revered, because he finally freed medicine from the shackles of magic, superstition, and the supernatural. He saw medicine as a rational science and for this, he is still widely accepted as the "Father of Western Medicine." Proof of that is the Hippocratic Oath which many medical schools require potential doctors to take, at one point during their studies. Although there are now new versions of this oath, the core of the documents are similar in that they deal with the treatment of patients, the respect for confidentiality and the passing of medical knowledge to the future generations of doctors.

Unfortunately most graduating students never learn, unless they study on their own, that Hippocrates was a holistic doctor in that he treated the whole patient and not just the disease. He saw the physician as the servant and facilitator of Nature. All medical treatment was aimed at enabling the natural resistance of the organism to withstand and overcome the disease and to bring about the recovery, health and harmony to the afflicted person.

In his own words: **"Everyone has a doctor in him or her; we just have to help it in it's work. The natural healing force within each of us is the greatest force in getting well."**

That's one powerful statement!

I thought: *"I have a doctor in me?, where? what is he talking about?"*

Then I pondered on these questions some more and it dawned on me that maybe the inner doctor he's referring to is our own immune system, that wonderful gift of nature that we receive from our mother, as we pass through the birth canal. It works arduously, 24/7, to protect us and bring physical harmony to our bodies. Whether we're awake or sleeping, it's fighting our battles against external and internal invaders (viruses, infections, toxins, etc.). And, according to Hippocrates, all it's asking us to do is help it and not hinder it, while it does it's work, so that we can experience wellbeing. It began to make sense to me!

How can we help the doctor within do it's work?

Well, then he goes on to say: **"Food should be our medicine and medicine our food."**

Could it be that simple? Was Hippocrates on the right track? Has modern medicine, with it's overwhelming dependence on chemical drugs and invasive procedures to cure disease, lost it's way. The growing mountain of evidence is showing that this indeed may be the case...as we head down a dark dead end street, where chronic diseases and premature death prevail?

T. Colin Campbell, Phd and author of the NYT bestseller "The China Study", calls the paradigm under which modern medicine operates, reductionism, where science looks for truth only in the smallest details, while entirely ignoring the big picture. The popular expression "can't see the forest for the trees" makes the point well, except that there's much more at stake here than just trees and forests.

I remember the old Indian fable about the six blind men attempting to describe an elephant. One feels the trunk and describes the elephant as a snake. Another feels the tusk and describes a spear, a third says the leg is a tree trunk, and so on. All of the explanations have merit, but each individual's conclusion doesn't describe the whole, which in this case is the elephant. Once we see the elephant then the separate findings make sense.

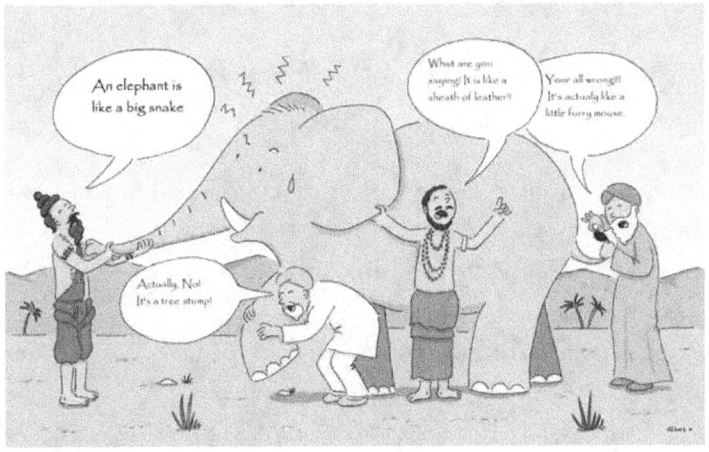

With regards to nutrition, reductionism has played a crucial part in the development of pharmaceutical drugs, with the accompanying side effects, and vitamin and mineral supplements to cure diseases...both multi-billion dollar industries. As a result, it becomes more and more difficult for us to accept real food as medicine.

Although considered the Father of Western Medicine, because of his holistic approach to health, one can see striking similarities between the system used by Hippocrates and Oriental medicine, where both consider the whole person and not just the disease.

Hopefully, one day doctors will accept and integrate the wisdom of Hippocrates into their practice. Then maybe we'll begin to see a reversal of the current trend towards an increase in chronic diseases and premature death.

Until that day happens, maybe now is a good time to start taking charge of our own health.

IN SEARCH OF THE WISE DOCTORS
PART 1

Previously, I quoted the Father of Medicine, Hippocrates:

"Everyone has a doctor in him or her; we just have to help it in it's work.
The natural healing force within each of us is the greatest force in getting well."

If we accept that statement, which I do, as a key to improving our health, then the next question I ask is "how can I find a doctor or health care provider that supports that? What Hippocrates is actually saying is that my body's defenses can pretty much deal with my health problems…if I give it the necessary support. I remember many years ago, my doctor told me that, generally speaking, of all the patients that come to see him, 90% of what ails them can be cured by their own body's defenses. 90% of the remaining 10%, I can help them with. Unfortunately, nothing can be done for the remaining 1%.

How easy is it to find a supporting and caring doctor? In my experience…not easy at all. I've been living in Mexico for more than 40 years and although I've been searching and asking around, I haven't even found one (maybe I'm too picky). It's not completely a doctor's fault because he or she is not really prepared to look at a person's health from a different perspective than from what they've learned. They are just not given the tools (i.e., nutrition classes, lifestyle changes) to support people who wish to prevent illness and disease…as the first line of offense, instead of just treating the symptoms. Instead, they are provided the tools (i.e., drugs and invasive procedures) for treating people when they are already sick. Unfortunately, and as you can imagine, the pharmaceutical industry has a big stake in the preparation of doctors. It is the main sponsor of medical schools in the U.S. and ,as a result, has a lot to say with regards to what a doctor studies. No wonder why our doctors

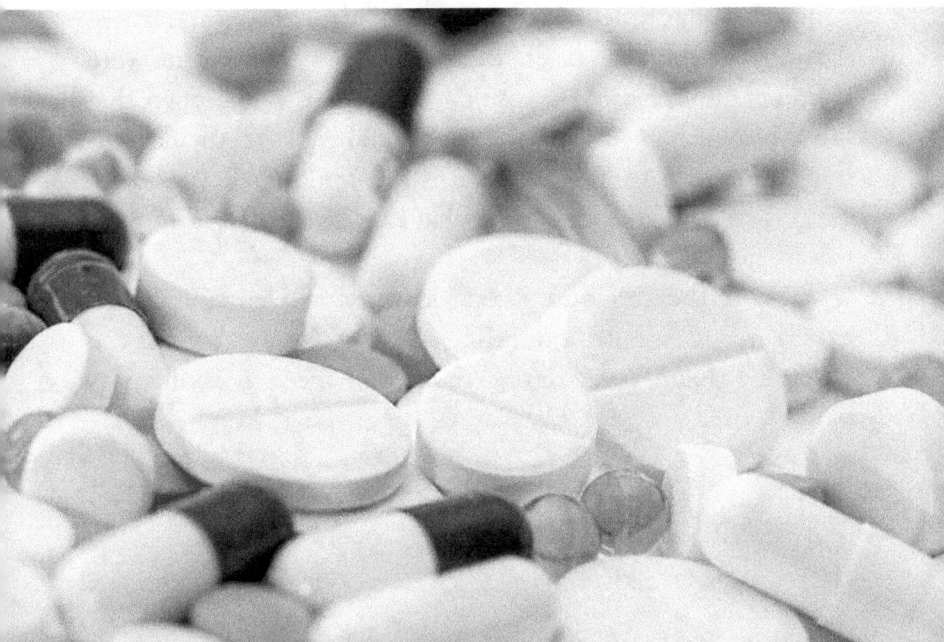

prescribe drugs for pretty much everything…of course, with all of the accompanying side effects.

So… what can we do?

Well, on the one hand, we can wait for the day when doctor's become educated and well informed on the subject of nutrition and it's relation to illness and disease, or we can search for "wise" doctors who can help us in our quest for disease prevention.

One of the definitions of wisdom I found is: "Knowledge that is gained by having many experiences in life and the ability to understand things that most other people can't."

HOW CAN WE DETERMINE IF A DOCTOR IS WISE?

Well, one way would be for the doctor to have once been a part of the medical establishment, only to become aware and convinced over time that the "accepted" treatments and cures, for most chronic diseases, were either not working or were counterproductive. As a result, said doctor would then distance him or herself from the traditional approach by becoming committed to finding alternative options that worked. They then could share with us what they've learned from their experiences.

Taking the above into consideration, as well as my own experience with nutrition during the past 7 years, for me the following doctors are among those that meet the criteria as being "wise."

Michael Greger, MD

Author of the NY Times best seller, "How Not to Die" and the founder of the extremely popular and informative http://www.nutritionfacts.org. All the proceeds from his books, website and speaking engagements are donated to charity.

Dr. Greger is a physician, and an internationally recognized speaker on nutrition, food safety, and public health issues. A founding member and Fellow of the American College of Lifestyle Medicine, Dr. Greger is licensed as a general practitioner specializing in clinical nutrition. Currently he proudly serves as the public health director at the Humane Society of the United States. He is a graduate of the Cornell University School of Agriculture and the Tufts University School of Medicine.

As a doctor he became aware of the growing evidence, published in some of the most prestigious medical journals in the world, that diet and lifestyle changes can indeed prevent and even reverse heart disease.

And, in his own words:

"Yet medical practice hardly changed. Why? Why were doctors still prescribing drugs and using Roto-Rooter-type procedures to just treat the symptoms of heart disease and to try to forestall what they chose to believe was inevitable – an early death?

This was my wake-up call. I opened my eyes to the depressing fact that there are other forces at work in medicine besides science. The U.S. health care system runs on a fee for service model in which doctors get paid for the pills and procedures they prescribe, rewarding quantity over quality. We (doctors) don't get reimbursed for time spent counseling our patients about the benefits of healthy eating. If doctors were instead paid for performance, there would be a financial incentive to treat the lifestyle causes of disease. Until the model of reimbursement changes, I don't expect great changes in medical care or medical education."

IN SEARCH OF THE WISE DOCTORS
PART 2

I had been a vegetarian since 1978, until my brother Arthur, who is in his 80s now, told me about the benefits that he was experiencing after four years on a whole food vegan diet. As a vegetarian I felt quite healthy…most of the time. However, during those 32 vegetarian years I remember that almost every year I would become ill a couple of times…with sore throats, coughing, nasal congestion, etc. Although I never had fevers, the uncomfortableness and pain would last up to 2 weeks. Changing from vegetarian to whole food vegan wasn't easy for me. My problem, which is the problem that most people have, was giving up dairy…especially cheese…especially pizza. I eventually accepted the challenge 7 years ago and haven't looked back since. The results: I haven't gotten sick during all this time. Living in San Miguel and because of the climate changes, almost all my friends would eventually become ill, to one degree or another. "Knock on wood", it still hasn't happened to me. As a result, I haven't had the need to see doctors. What sparked my search for "wise" doctors was when my brother suggested that I check out Dr. John McDougall's website.

So, next on my list of "wise doctors":

Dr. John McDougall:

Because he has on one of the largest collections of nutrition archives in the United States and has been following a whole food vegan diet since the 1970s I felt that I could rely on his information. I also found that he's very accessible in that he responds to questions through his contact page. I have consulted him on various occasions and he or a member of his team usually responds within the same day. In 2017 he started a free weekly online webinar where he covers different themes on nutrition and answers questions from the attendees. At the present time the webinars are on Mondays. You can register on his website: http://www.drmcdougall.com.

A physician and nutrition expert who teaches better health through whole plant food cuisine, Dr. McDougall has been studying, writing, and speaking out about the effects of nutrition on disease for over 40 years. He believes that people should look and feel great for a lifetime. Unfortunately, many people unknowingly compromise their health through poor dietary habits. One of my favorite sayings of his is: "People love to hear good things about their bad habits."

Dr. McDougall has cared for thousands of patients for almost 4 decades. His program not only promotes a broad range of dramatic and lasting health benefits but, most importantly, can also reverse serious illnesses including high blood pressure, heart disease, diabetes and others, all without the use of drugs. He is the author of "The Healthiest Diet on the Planet" as well as several other books.

Dr. Caldwell Esselstyn

Previously I wrote about Beatriz, a friend of my wife and I, who had undergone cuadruple bypass heart surgery 7 years ago and a year later suffered complications. Although the cardiologists pretty much gave up hope on her recovery, thanks to my nutrition suggestions, today she is still alive and "kicking." It was Dr. Esselstyn's NY Times bestseller, "Prevent and Reverse Heart Disease" that had a lot to do with her acceptance of the challenge to change her eating habits. It is also the book behind Bill Clinton's life changing diet.

Dr. Esselstyn has been associated with the Cleveland Clinic since 1968. During that time, he has served as President of the Staff and as a member of the Board of Governors. He chaired the Clinic's Breast Cancer Task Force and headed its Section of Thyroid and Parathyroid Surgery. He is a Fellow of the American College of Cardiology.

In 1991, Dr. Esselstyn served as President of the American Association of Endocrine Surgeons, That same year he organized the first National Conference on the Elimination of Coronary Artery Disease, which was held in Tucson, Arizona. In 1997, he chaired a follow-up conference, the Summit on Cholesterol and Coronary Disease, which brought together more than 500 physicians and health-care workers in Lake Buena Vista, Florida. In April, 2005, Dr. Esselstyn became the first recipient of the Benjamin Spock Award for Compassion in Medicine. He received the Distinguished Alumnus Award from the Cleveland Clinic Alumni Association in 2009. In September 2010, he received the Greater Cleveland Sports

Hall of Fame Award. Dr. Esselstyn received the 2013 Deerfield Academy Alumni Association Heritage Award In Recognition of Outstanding Achievement & Service, and the 2013 Yale University George H.W. Bush '48 Lifetime of Leadership Award. Dr. Esselstyn has also received the 2015 Plantrician Project Luminary Award, the Case Western Reserve University School of Medicine 2016 Distinguished Alumni Award, and the American College of Lifestyle Medicine 2016 Lifetime Achievement Award. http://www.dresselstyn.com.

Doctors, Drugs and the Medical Profession

IN SEARCH OF THE WISE DOCTORS
PART 3

Finding "wise doctors has been very important for me on during my whole food vegan journey. It has taken me several years of reading, investigating and experiencing personally the benefits of this lifestyle to finally come up with a correct list of doctors… that works for me. The knowledge I've acquired during this time has enabled me to solve my own health problems and given me the confidence to share with the public what I have been learning.

For me the bottom line is that, before you embark on a new nutrition journey or in fact any new journey, each step you take should make sense. If it doesn't then you might be advancing on shaky ground and vulnerable to different ideas and opinions from others that can easily cause confusion and take you off your chosen path. If you closely adhere to a whole food vegan diet, within weeks you should be experiencing the following benefits:

- **A noticeable increase in energy**
- **A gradual loss of weight**
- **An overall feeling of wellbeing**
- **The realization that following the Standard American Diet is a definite health risk and is not taking you where you want to go.**

The first influential book I read on my journey was "The China Study", by T. Colin Campbell which, released in 2005, has already sold over 2 million books worldwide. The revised edition, containing a lot of new information, was released in 2015. Between these two books came the extraordinary "Whole" which explains, in great detail, where and how the western medical profession has gone wrong.

T. Colin Campbell, PhD
For decades T. Colin Campbell, PhD has been at the forefront of nutrition education and research. Dr. Campbell's expertise and scientific interests encompass relationships between diet and diseases and particularly the relationship between animal protein as a cause of cancer. His legacy, the China Project, is one of the most comprehensive studies of health and nutrition ever conducted. The New York Times has recognized the study as the "Grand Prix of epidemiology", which is the study of the distribution of health and disease in different populations, as

well as the application of the specific study to the control of health problems.

Dr. Campbell has conducted original research both in laboratory experiments and in large-scale human studies; He has received over 70 grant-years of peer-reviewed research funding (mostly with the National Institute of Health), served on grant review panels of multiple funding agencies, actively participated in the development of national and international nutrition policy, authored over 300 research papers and given hundreds of lectures around the world.

He was trained at Cornell University (M.S., Ph.D.) and MIT (Research Associate) in nutrition, biochemistry and toxicology. Dr. Campbell spent 10 years on the faculty of Virginia Tech's Department of Biochemistry and Nutrition before returning to Cornell in 1975 where he presently holds his Endowed Chair as the Jacob Gould Schurman Professor Emeritus of Nutritional Biochemistry in the Division of Nutritional Sciences. http://www.nutritionstudies.org.

Dr. Neal Barnard

Neal Barnard, M.D., F.A.C.C., is an adjunct associate professor of medicine at the George Washington University School of Medicine and Health Sciences in Washington, D.C., president of the Physicians Committee for Responsible Medicine, and founder of Barnard Medical Center.

Dr. Barnard is a fellow of the American College of Cardiology, the 2016 recipient of the American College of Lifestyle Medicine's Trailblazer Award, and has led numerous research studies investigating the effects of diet on diabetes, body weight, and chronic pain, including a groundbreaking study of dietary interventions in type 2 diabetes, funded by the National Institutes of Health. Dr. Barnard has authored more than 70 scientific publications as well as 18 books, including the New York Times best-sellers "Power Foods for the Brain", "21-Day Weight Loss Kickstart", the USA Today best- seller "Dr. Barnard's Program for Reversing Diabetes" and his latest, "The Cheese Trap."

As president of the Physicians Committee, Dr. Barnard leads programs advocating for preventive medicine, good nutrition, and higher ethical standards in research. Recently, the Physicians Committee sponsored a new program in hospitals around the USA, calling for major changes in the menus of the foods being served. As a result, more than 200,000 US doctors are supporting the addition of more fruits and vegetables and the elimination of processed meats, which are classified by the World Health Organization, as cancer causing and in the same category as cigarettes. Dr. Bernard hosts four PBS television programs on nutrition and health and is frequently called on by news programs to discuss issues related to nutrition and research. http://www.pcrm.org

THE BENEFITS VS THE RISKS OF TAKING PRESCRIPTION MEDICINES

A friend of mine, with heart problems, had gone through open heart surgery seven years ago. She recently mentioned to me that she was having difficulty breathing. Her cardiologist advised her of a new drug that was now available, that was helping lots of people who were experiencing similar breathing problems. She became very interested in this new hope for relieving her symptoms but was concerned about possible side effects. As she had done on previous occasions she asked me to check out online, the possible side effects...which I did. What I found out was that one of side effects could actually produce the very symptom that she wanted to avoid. I told her about my findings and she still decided to take the risk and go ahead with the drug. She made her decision after weighing the benefits against the risks.

Why am I telling you this?
Well, a few days ago I went to my dentist to have a tooth extracted. He told me that I needed to take an antibiotic in order to prevent a possible infection. This was to be done for seven days, beginning the day before the extraction. Of course, he asked me if I was allergic to any antibiotics and I told him that I was not. Anyway, I bought 7 days worth of the medicine and had already taken 3 of the prescribed 14 tablets when, while walking, I felt a sharp pain behind my right knee, accompanied by the sensation of a tight tendon pull, in back of the knee. It was something that one would expect following excessive exercise. It was a strange and uncomfortable feeling. The next day I went out to do my usual walking exercise and noticed that the pain and pulling had gotten worse. I thought that stretching out the tendon would be a good way to "loosen" things up. To my surprise, not only did that not help, but I felt a second pull, accompanied by pain, on the back of my other leg, above the heel. I had to slow down and even completely

stop in my tracks, because of the pain and pulling of what I assumed were 2 tendons. "What's going on here"?, Then the thought came to me…"maybe it would be wise to check out the side effects of the drug I was taking." So, I went online and checked it out…and here's what part of the "warning" read:

Taking levofloxacin increases the risk that you will develop tendinitis (swelling of a fibrous tissue that connects a bone to a muscle) or have a tendon rupture (tearing of a fibrous tissue that connects a bone to a muscle) during your treatment or for up to several months afterward. These problems may affect tendons in your shoulder, your hand, the back of your ankle, or in other parts of your body. Tendinitis or tendon rupture may happen to people of any age, but the risk is highest in people over 60 years of age.

The warnings finish with:

Talk to your doctor about the risks of taking levofloxacin.

I must confess that I screwed up because of a lack of consciousness. Although I always tell people to read the side effects before taking a prescription medicine, in this case I didn't do that. It just didn't occur to me. After all…how dangerous could an antibiotic be?

For so many of us, we blindly tend to trust our doctor's advice, so much so, that we don't ask questions, when we should, or we're simply afraid to confront him or her, with our doubts. After all…what do we know? We forget that they're human beings just like us and, just like us, they make mistakes. Maybe, that's why, every year in the United States, prescription drug side effects kill over 200,000 people. On a list of causes of death, that would put it at #3, behind Heart Disease and Cancer and ahead of Respiratory Diseases and Accidents. And that doesn't include other damages that may not kill us but could seriously affect our lives and the lives of our loved ones. And the sad thing is that doctors' rarely have to answer for their mistakes...because they have nobody to answer to.

The FDA stance regarding prescription drug side effects!

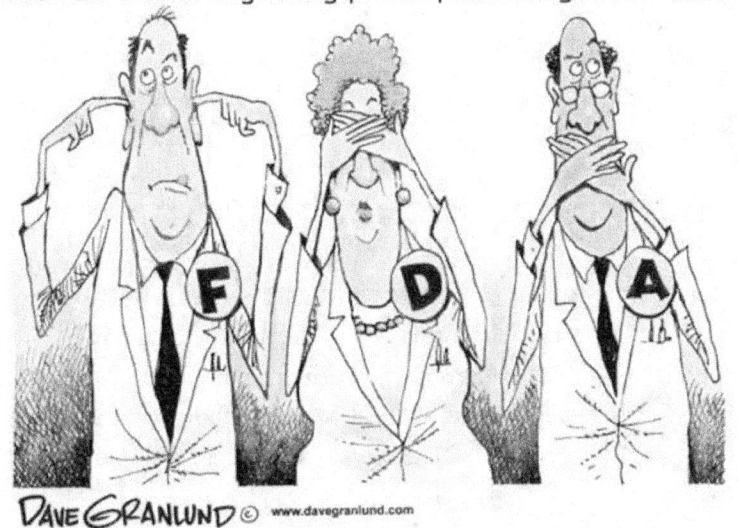

DAVE GRANLUND © www.davegranlund.com

In order to make a conscious decision we need to have sufficient information...so that we can make the right choice. In the case of my friend, once she became aware of the benefits as well as the risks, she could then weigh both sides and decide whether the benefits are worth the risks. If we are only told by our doctors about the benefits then our choice cannot be conscious. When we see a a drug being promoted on TV, we are told about the possible side effects. I listen to the ads and find it hard to believe that someone would actually take that drug. But at least people are being given the pros and the cons, so that they can make a personal decision.

For some reason that transparency which we see on the TV is not being afforded to us by so many doctors. We are not being told about possible side effects of the prescription drugs we take. For that reason, we need to assume that responsibility by checking the information online. If we don't, then we are gambling with our lives, increasing the possibility that, one day, we may become part of that 200,000 statistic.

WHAT'S THE 3RD LEADING CAUSE OF DEATH – Revised

What most people don't know is that the medical profession, including doctors, drugs and hospitals, is the 3rd leading cause of death in the United States…. producing over 400,000 annual deaths, only exceeded by heart disease (600,000+) and cancer (600,000+) (Journal of the American Medical Association).

The reasons for this are:

- *Patients not following medication indications*
- *Wrong medications given to patients*
- *Infections acquired in hospitals*
- *Unnecessary surgeries*
- *Errors in surgery*
- *Prescription drug side effects (over 200,000)*

This is well documented information that members of the medical profession are aware of and we are not. Why are we not aware of this data? Is this being kept from us? Well, for one thing, imagine if you had this this information. Might you not look at doctors, hospitals and prescription drugs from a different perspective and with more scrutiny?

Now, don't get me wrong. I never underestimate the important role of doctors. For example, their value is obvious when it comes to:

- **Diagnosis**
- **Repairing fractures**
- **Healing wounds**
- **Curing infections with medication**
- **Relieving pain and discomfort with medication**
- **Removing the symptoms of illness and chronic disease**
- **Saving lives through chemotherapy, surgery and radiation**

However, when it comes to preventing and even reversing chronic diseases, before they actually happen, the great majority of doctors are not prepared for that, simply because that was not a priority of their education.

So, if that statement is true, what can we do to prevent and reverse diseases? First of all, we need to accept that the solution is mainly up to us…that we're the ones that will make a difference. That we're the ones that need to empower ourselves with the responsibility of doing all we can do to remain healthy.

It's so important to remember that our body is our friend. It's objective is to be in harmony and when it is, we feel good... with no pain or discomfort. We feel so comfortable that we don't even notice it and we "know" that this physical state is the way it's supposed to be. Yet, to achieve this state of well-being our bodies are involved in a constant war (24/7) with external and internal invaders that are trying to dethrone it's protective army...the immune system. The results: Illness and disease, whether it be the flu, the common cold or a more serious threat. So, while we're dealing with our life's circumstances and problem solving, we are oblivious to the battles that our "friend" is constantly involved in...just to keep us healthy.

So, our responsibility actually is to help our body fight it's "battles" by not getting in it's way...and by adopting healthy lifestyle habits such as exercising, avoiding stress and most important...making **plant powered foods** the foundation of our health. If we do this then we will most probably reduce our dependency on the medical profession, to tell us what we need to do and rely more on our own understanding? Think of some of the perks! **Less worry and fear about getting sick, feeling healthier and with more energy, reaching one's ideal weight, having the potencial of living a longer, healthier life and spending less money on medical care.**

SCREENING FOR CANCERS – Mammograms

October is Breast Cancer Awareness Month in many countries throughout the world. Here in San Miguel de Allende,

Mexico it's no different. The slogan is **"Early Detection is The Solution."** Wait a minute! Shouldn't the slogan be **"Prevention is The Solution?"** Detection means that you already got it…and chances are you've had it for many years… even decades…but didn't know it, until now, when the cancer has already reached a size that is detectable, either by self-examination or a machine.

Dr. Michael Greger, author of the New York Times Best Seller, "How Not to Die", states:
"The breast cancer you may feel one day as a lump in the shower may have started 20 years before. We now suspect that all the epithelial cancers— breast, colon, lung, pancreas, prostate, ovarian—the ones that cause the vast majority of cancer deaths— may have been growing for up to 20 years or more. By the time it's picked up, it may have already been growing, maturing, scheming, for years— acquiring hundreds of new survival-of-the-fittest mutations to grow even quicker and to better undermine our immune system. So-called "early detection," like by mammogram, is really, really, really late detection."

On a more personal note, during World War 2, my dad was stationed at the Brooklyn Navy Yard. His duty was to paint the lower decks of ships, including the Queen Mary. At that time asbestos was widely used for heat resistance and electrical insulation on ships. Unfortunately, no connection was made between asbestos exposure and cancer. That was in 1943. In 1986 he experienced chest pains and was diagnosed with Mesothelioma, a lung cancer caused by asbestos. That cancer was 43 years in the making!

According to the Department and Research Unit of General Practice, Institute of Public Health, University of Copenhagen, Copenhagen, Denmark:

"The balance between benefits and harms is delicate for cancer screening programs. By attending screening with mammography some women will avoid dying from breast cancer or receive less aggressive treatment. But many more women will be over- diagnosed, receive needless treatment, have a false-positive result, or live more years as a patient with breast cancer. Systematic reviews of the randomized trials have shown that for every 2000 women invited for mammography screening throughout 10 years, only 1 will have her life prolonged. In addition, 10 healthy women will be over- diagnosed with breast cancer and will be treated unnecessarily. Furthermore, more than 200 women will experience substantial psychosocial distress for months because of false-positive findings. Regular breast self-examination does not reduce breast cancer mortality, but doubles the number of biopsies, and it therefore cannot be recommended. It is not clear whether screening with mammography does more good than harm. Women invited to screening should be informed according to the best available evidence."

In other words, with all the hullabaloo surrounding National Breast Cancer Awareness Month (NBCAM) and the importance of getting tested, women are not being informed enough about the harm that can result from screening. Unfortunately, because of the people's trust and faith in Doctors and the medical profession, individual decisions are often made blindly, because all of the facts are not available. Decisions are faith-based instead of evidence-based.

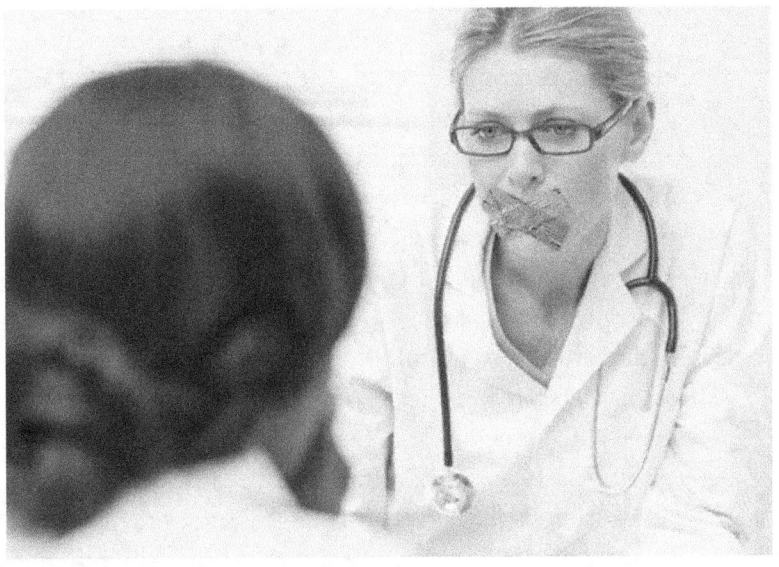

BREAST CANCER – Big business?

National Breast Cancer Awareness Month was established in 1985 as a partnership between the American Cancer Society and the pharmaceutical division of **Imperial Chemical Industries** (now part of AstraZeneca, a leading manufacturer of oncology drugs). It's the 5th largest pharmaceutical company in the world…with branches in more than 100 countries. This might lead us to the conclusion that breast cancer is big business and mammography is one of it's primary profit centers. Since the industries goal is to maintain and increase profits it would be beneficial for them to downplay the risks and keep women uninformed.

Below are a few key points for women to consider when choosing whether or not to undergo a mammogram screening:

1. For every 2,000 women receiving mammograms, only ONE would have her life extended at all. TEN women, though, might be harmed with chemotherapy, radiation or mastectomies.

2. **Mammograms expose your body to ionized radiation that may cause cancer** by triggering mutations and other genetic damage as well as cause normal cells to become malignant.

3. A newer type of mammogram touted to be much better at detecting breast cancers called **tomosynthesis** takes a 3D image of the breast. You definitely want to avoid this type of mammogram because it uses three times more radiation than the standard type.

4. Mammography also compresses your breasts tightly, and often painfully, damaging the breast tissue which could lead to a lethal spread of cancerous cells, should they exist.

5. Dr. Charles B. Simone, a former clinical associate in immunology and pharmacology at the National Cancer Institute, said, "Mammograms increase the risk for developing breast cancer and raise the risk of spreading or metastasizing an existing growth."

6. Aside from the radiation risks, mammograms carry a first time false positive rate of up to 6 percent. False positives can lead to expensive repeat screenings and often results in unnecessary chemotherapy and radiation treatments and surgeries.

7. 80% of the 1.6 million breast biopsies done each year in the United States, because of a suspicious mammography, are negative.

8. The problem with mammograms is that they often detect "cancer" that would never spread or do any harm if left untreated. It's called "stage zero" cancer. **It can be regressed by simple lifestyle changes and without any medical treatment.**

9. *The New England Journal of Medicine* has pointed to approximately 1.3 million cases of misdiagnosed breast cancer, which shows that **mammograms are leading millions of women astray, making them think they have cancer when they really don't.**

10. Just thinking you may have breast cancer, when you really do not, focuses your mind on fear and disease, and is actually enough to trigger an illness in your body. So a false positive on a mammogram, or an unnecessary biopsy, can really be damaging.

CONCLUSIONS:

- Self – Examination and mammograms can only detect cancers that have had many years even decades to develop. A cancer just doesn't pop up.
- Since mammograms can do more harm than good, it's important to demand all of the facts from your health care practitioner before making a decision.
- Since the Medical Profession is not telling us the whole truth, in order to make a conscious choice, women need to be more proactive and investigate on their own whether or not to get a mammogram.

- Since cancer "prevention" and not "detection" is the best solution... to avoid this disease, as well as other chronic diseases, it is incumbent upon each one of us to make healthy lifestyle changes...before it's too late.

SCREENING FOR CANCER -The Prostate Specific Antigen (PSA) test

I hope that for those people who follow my Facebook page it has become obvious that my intentions have always been to provide cutting edge information on health and nutrition. The topics I choose are supported by the results of my own experience on a Whole Food Plant Based diet during these past 8+ years as well as the latest fact based nutrition research. You the reader may not agree to all the information I include on my posts but I believe that what's most important is to be well informed. Only then can a person have the best opportunity to make more conscious choices regarding his or her health.

THE DOCTOR – PATIENT RELATIONSHIP

There are basically 2 situations when we get to see a doctor and become a patient. The first one is when we're feeling ill. In that case we take the initiative and make an appointment. The second scenario is when doctors decide to come looking for you and me and one of the most successful ways is via cancer screening. We may be feeling fantastic and enjoying our lives... our family...our hobbies and not thinking about doctors at all. All of a sudden there's a campaign...breast screening for women and prostate screening for men. Out of fear, worry or concern, we somehow convince ourselves that participating in one of these screenings is the right thing to do.

Screening for prostate cancer began in the early 1990s with the Prostate Specific Antigen Test (PSA) and it's popularity has grown exponentially since then as more and more men undergo the test every year. Campaigns have been so effective that about 75 percent of men in the USA have had a routine PSA test.

So, What's The Evidence?

Dr. Otis Brawley is the Chief Medical and Scientific Officer for the American Cancer Society. He's responsible for promoting the goals of cancer prevention, early detection, and quality treatment through cancer research and education.

About himself he says, *"I have never had a PSA and do not desire one."* He wrote in the journal Cancer (published on behalf of the American Cancer Society), *"The benefits of screening and early detection, although theoretically possible, are yet unknown, whereas the risks and harms of screening and resultant treatment are definite."* He continued, *"Although it (screening) may truly cure a few men who need to be cured, this benefit may be achieved at the cost of causing a large number of men with prostate cancer to undergo unnecessary treatment and resultant illness."*

In other words, when it comes to screening, Dr. Brawley continues to have many reservations about its value in saving lives, as well its role leading to over-diagnosis and unnecessary treatment. He says that he has known for years about the lack of medical evidence for screening and that despite that, most men with PSAs greater than 4

would receive a biopsy, and if it revealed prostate cancer, they were told that they needed to be treated soon, with younger men usually directed towards surgery and older men towards radiation therapy.

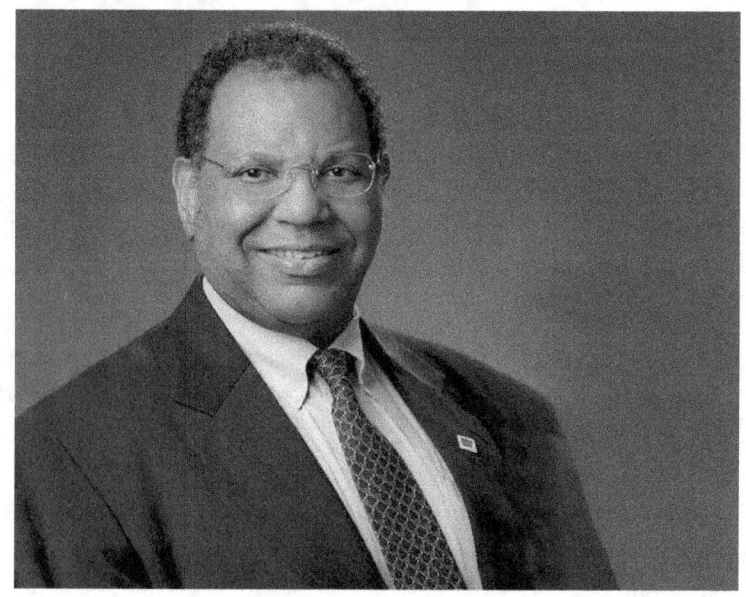

Dr. Otis Brawly

"Hospitals and clinics started business plans to get into community screening that were all about money before we had any evidence that prostate cancer screening could save lives," he said.

The **NATIONAL HEALTH SERVICE of the United Kingdom** does not recommend the PSA test and always informs it's patients about the pros and cons:

PROS:

- It may reassure you if the test result is normal
- It can find early signs of cancer, meaning you can get treated early
- PSA testing may reduce your risk of dying if you do have cancer

CONS:

- It can miss cancer and provide false reassurance
- It may lead to unnecessary worry and medical tests when there's no cancer
- It cannot tell the difference between slow-growing and fast-growing cancers
- It may make you worry by finding a slow-growing cancer that may never cause any problems

According to a 2014 Consumer Reports, developed in cooperation with the AMERICAN ACADEMY OF FAMILY PHYSICIANS:

Up to 25% of men with high PSAs may have prostate cancer, depending on age and PSA level. But most of these cancers do not cause problems. It is common for older men to have some cancer cells in their prostate glands. These cancers are usually slow to grow. They are not likely to spread beyond the prostate. They usually don't cause symptoms, or death. Studies show that routine PSA tests of 1,000 men ages 55 to 69 prevent only one prostate cancer death.

If your PSA is not normal, you will probably have a biopsy. The doctor puts a needle through the wall of the rectum and into the prostate to take a few samples. Biopsies can be painful and cause bleeding. Men can get serious infections from biopsies, and they may need hospital care.

Surgery or radiation are the usual treatments for prostate cancer. They can do more harm than good. Treatment can cause serious complications, such as heart attacks, blood clots in the legs or lungs, or even death. In addition, 40 men out of 1,000 will become impotent or incontinent from treatment.

Even the MAYO CLINIC states:

Neither the PSA test nor the digital rectal exam provides enough information for your doctor to diagnose prostate cancer. Abnormal results in these tests may lead your doctor to recommend a prostate biopsy.

So What Are We Supposed to Do?

Even with all the controversy and conflicting evidence…the screening campaigns continue for breast and prostate cancer. These campaigns never inform us of the pros and cons of the tests or give us sufficient information so that we can make the right decision or at least have a discussion with our doctor or health care professional.

From my perspective, the best action is to be pro-active so that we don't have to worry or depend on cancer screenings that can have so much downside. The right path to health is to make the best lifestyle choices in order to prevent these cancers…not to wait until we're struggling to survive.

Of all Possible Lifestyle Choices, why a Whole Food, Plant Based diet?

According to Dr. Michael Greger, author of the NY Times Best Seller, "How Not to Die."

"If you look around the world, there are huge differences in prostate cancer rates. In the USA the rates are up to a hundred times higher than some places in Asia, for example. And, it's not just genetic; within one generation of coming to the U.S., cancer rates shoot up, and then their grandkids end up with the same rates as the population they now live in. A whole range of "lifestyle factors" have been looked at, but diet appears to have the greatest influence. Specifically, "the consumption of meat and dairy...appears to increase risk, and consumption of plant... foods appears to decrease risk."

5

ARE WE BEING DUPED?

"Don't eat anything your great, great grandmother wouldn't recognize as food. There are a great many food-like items in the supermarket your ancestors wouldn't recognize as food. Stay away from these."

Prof. Michael Pollan,
author of "The Omnivore's Dilemma"

HEALTH CARE OR DISEASE CARE?

Until 8 years ago I was a faithful paying client of Health Care insurance here in Mexico. The insurance covered pretty much any illness I could possibly contract. Unfortunately, once I reached the age of 65 (I'm now 76), the cost of the policy began increasing a whopping 25% annually. To compensate for the constant increases, I had to increase the deductible. Needless to say it was a vicious cycle that I decided to break 8 years ago. It was also around that time that I switched from a

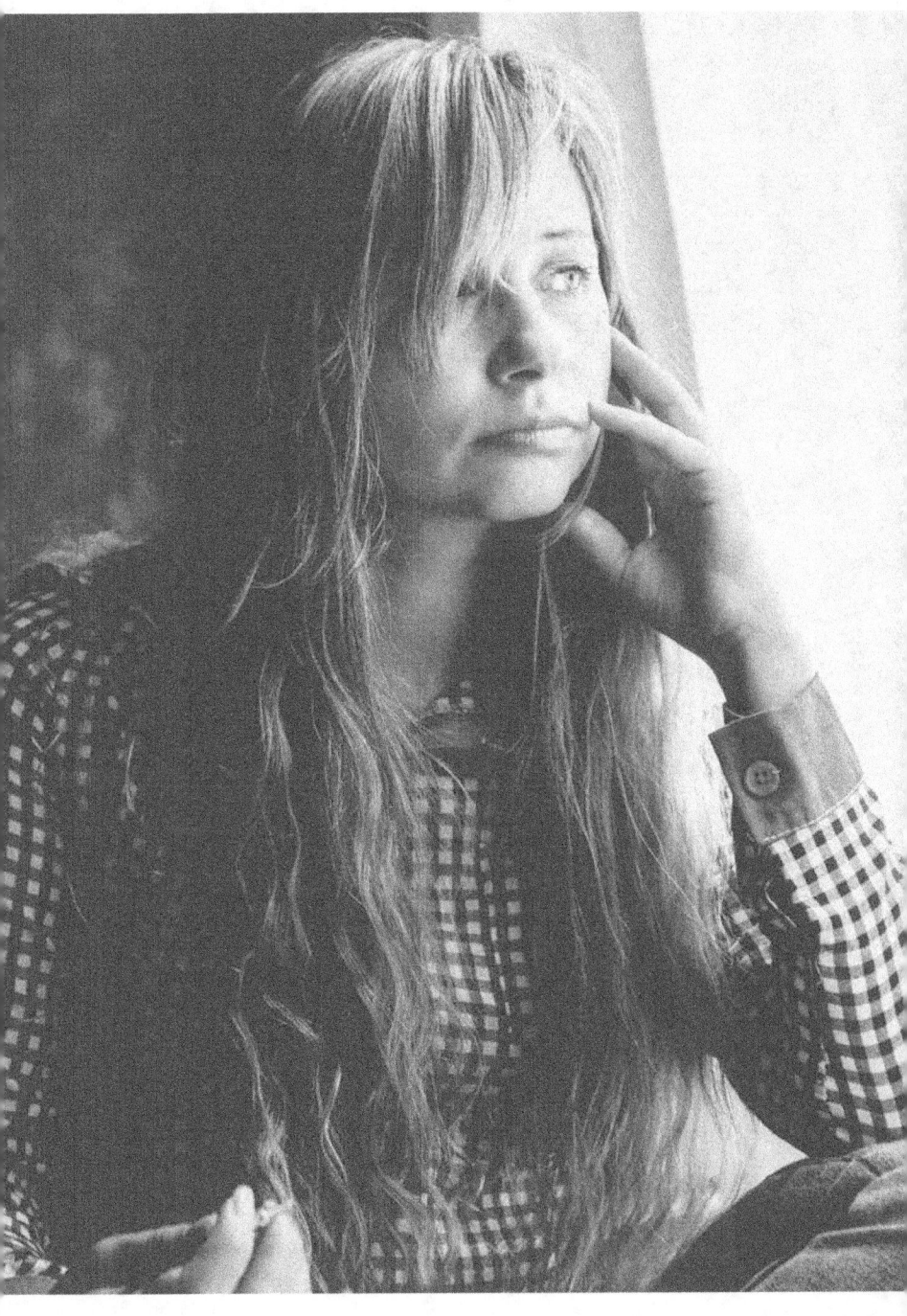

vegetarian to a Whole Food Plant Based Diet (WFPB). That meant sacrificing dairy products, apart from the meat that I had given up 32 years before. To be honest, it wasn't easy, especially since, as a Mexican resident for 40+ years, eliminating quesadillas (tortillas filled with cheese) from my diet, was for me a monumental decision. You see, quesadillas is as "Mexican pie" as pizza is "American pie." I understood, at that time, that cancelling the insurance would be a gamble and thoughts of "what if I get very sick" often rumbled through my mind. I did have Mexican Social Security…but only for emergencies. I decided that to give myself the best chance to stay healthy and to avoid costly doctors and expensive hospitals was to boost my immune system by eating WFPB foods. As the years past I became more confident in my decision to follow a healthier lifestyle, especially since I've been able to avoid getting ill during these past 8 years. I don't "knock on wood" because I don't think it's luck that has protected me all these years…but what has…are the following healthy lifestyle changes that I made:

1. **Consuming Whole Plant Based Foods (I believe this must be the Foundation of any healthy lifestyle)**
2. **Doing Moderate Exercise 5 Days per Week**
3. **Avoiding excessive Stress**
4. **Getting a Good Night Sleep**
5. **Having an inner purpose**

In the United States, Health Care costs have skyrocketed during the past few decades, so much so, that even with the

Affordable Care Act (Obamacare), close to 30,000,000 citizens still don't have health insurance...mostly because they can't afford it. Also, the number of annual bankruptcies resulting from people unable to pay their medical bills is calculated at 4000+. These statistics are discomforting, to say the least, especially when you take a look at other developed countries that have either Universal and/or Free Health care (i.e., Britain, France, Germany, Canada, Japan, Spain, Norway, Sweden and Australia). There...everyone is covered and there are 0 bankruptcies. Yes, we can argue that the health care in these countries is of inferior quality...yet globally, *the World Health Organization ranks the U.S. Health care system a distant #37 (France is #1). The measurements for the rankings include life expectancy, infant mortality, hospital beds per capita, medical care expenditures per person and fewer deaths related to surgical or medical mistakes.*

Maybe one day the United States will have Universal and/or Free Health Care but, from my perspective, that's not the main problem nor the solution. Why, because **Government run Health Care systems, regardless of the country, focus on treating the symptoms of diseases and rarely on disease prevention or reversal.** That's why the title of this post reads...Health Care or Disease Care. People are not only, not informed or educated on how to prevent and/or reverse diseases, but are often denied factual and research based information that could help them consider their options and make conscious health decisions. As a result, there's a constant dependence on doctor visits, pharmaceutical medications and medical interventions, prescribed for certain diseases that often can be reversed through simple lifestyle changes (i.e., Type 2 diabetes, Heart Disease, Hypertension, Obesity, etc.).

One example of information that is being denied to U.S. Citizens is found within the government's annual list of top ten causes of death, published by The U.S. Centers for Disease Control and Prevention. What is not included is information revealed in 2016 by the prestigious Journal of the American Medical Association. It stated that physician error, medication error, adverse events from surgery and side effects from drugs were killing 250,000 people per year. Maybe that's just another number to us but, when put in context, **it makes the health care system the third leading cause of death in the United States, behind only cancer and heart disease.**

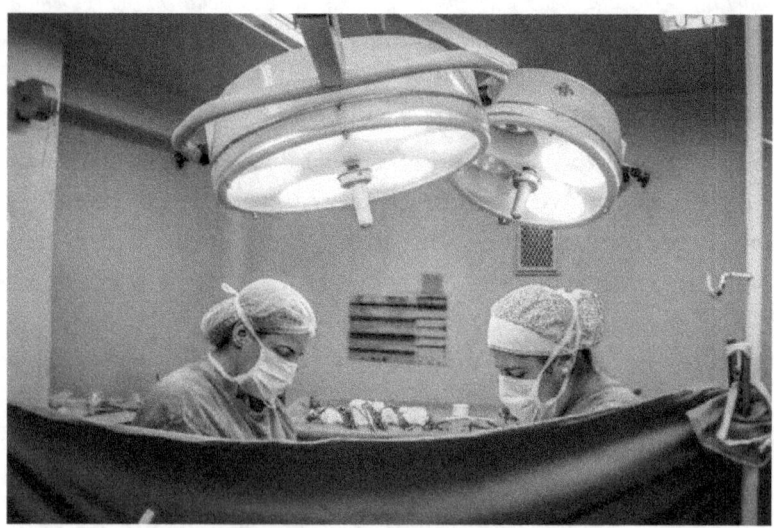

Medical mistakes kill over 250,000 Americans each year. If they were a disease, they would be the 3rd leading cause of death in the US.

That's pretty astounding information, yet unless you do some research on your own, you'll never see it on the official charts showing the Leading Causes of Death. Can you imagine why we're being denied that information? Well, maybe with that information we would be more cautious with regards to the medications that are prescribed or with a procedure that our doctor is recommending. With the right information we become "informed" and that can lead to more options and an opportunity to make the right choices.

WHERE CAN WE FIND THE BEST HEALTH CARE SYSTEM?

The healthiest people on the planet, who also live the longest, rarely suffer and die from the Chronic Diseases that plague people on the Standard American Diet, which is heavily biased towards meat, dairy, eggs and processed and refined foods. They live in rural China and Japan, parts of Africa and the Blue Zones (Okinawa Japan, Sardinia; Italy, Nicoya, Costa Rica, Icaria, Greece and The Seventh Day Adventists in Loma Linda California). They rely on their own personal health care system, that not only treats the symptoms of illness and disease, but also works 24/7 on prevention and reversal. That system is not sponsored by any government but is found within the body of every person on the planet…and it's free! *However, for it to function, we need to pay more attention to it's needs, to care for it and feed it the foods that it thrives on. What has worked for me for the past 8 years are the 4 points I mention above. It's similar to the lifestyle of the healthiest people. It's really very simple and rewarding…with the prize being optimal health and an overall feeling of wellbeing.*

CAN NUTRITION STUDIES BE TRUSTED?
PART 1

How can we know whether or not to believe what we read or hear...on nutrition and it's connection to health and wellbeing? After all there is so much conflicting information floating around out there...on social media.

Is coffee good for us...and how many cups per day? What about wine? Are potatoes fattening? Does soy have hormones? What about so called "heart healthy" oils? Is gluten free for everyone etc., etc., etc.? The list can go on and on.

Why is there so much confusion that sometimes prevents us from making the correct healthy choices for ourselves and our loved ones?

For one thing we may not know or understand that there are influential and powerful corporations and institutions that we're up against...that are more interested in their own welfare and survival than our own personal health... and, as a consequence, would do literally anything in order to make sure that we continue to consume their products. How powerful and influential are they? Well just to give you an example, we just have to go back to the mid 1900s when Big Tobacco was in control, mostly through the press and TV. Everybody smoked then. After all, if famous actors, athletes and doctors smoked...what could be wrong with that? At that time we were never given the chance to question whether it was a healthy habit or not. This was going on even though, since the 1940s, 1000s of studies were already showing the link between smoking and lung cancer. During that time millions would die from the disease...until the Surgeon

General finally published the warning in 1976. That was 42 years ago and, although cigarette sales have gone down, 30 million still smoke and 6,000,000 die each year from tobacco related diseases. Will the cigarette companies quit? Why should they...as long as the profits keep rolling in? Now, what is in vogue is electronic vapor cigarettes (E- cigarettes). Considered somewhat safer than regular cigarettes because of less heat and chemicals, it's goal is to keep the nicotine addiction going, especially among young people...the hook being "flavored" vapor. As a multi-billion dollar industry they developed an infallible strategy, based on constant advertising, skewed studies and the support of paid celebrities, politicians and representatives of the medical profession. Since we have a tendency believe what we read, especially if it's repeated again and again, we believed then that smoking was OK...even healthy. We were hoodwinked for decades. Now we know the connection, but at what price? 30,000,000 in the U.S. still remain addicted to nicotine, via one product or another.

FAST FORWARD TO THE PRESENT!
If we naively fell for false information and advertising 70 years ago, isn't it possible that there are certain organizations that are applying similar tactics utilized by Big Tobacco, that worked extremely well...to get us to consume their products? Why I single out these following institutions and corporations is because they are valued in the billions, giving them lots of power and influence over us and also because of their highly questionable interest in our personal health and wellbeing.

Through the manipulation of scientific studies and publicity their strategies are to confuse the public and to introduce doubt…not unlike the goals of the tobacco industry:

- **The Pharmaceutical Industry** – Drug sales, including dangerous side effects, are valued globally at one trillion dollars.
- **The American Heart Association**, The American Cancer Society and the American Diabetes Association – Their sponsors include the following food companies… all questionable foods for people with chronic diseases.

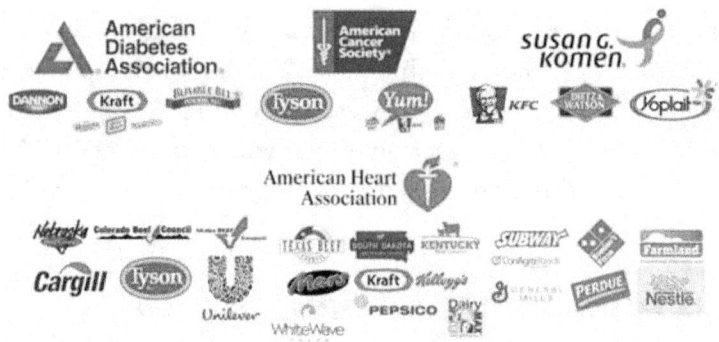

- **The Agricultural Industry** – Factory Farms satisfy our craving for meat, that lacks the fiber, antioxidants and phytonutrients, so essential for optimal health.
- **The Dairy Industry** – The Dairy = Healthy Calcium myth has been going on for decades.

- **The Egg Industry** – Food with highest cholesterol (1 egg = 200gms with 300mg being the Recommended Daily Requirement).
- **The Medical Profession** – 3rd leading cause of death in the U.S. (hospital and physician errors, drug misuse and side effects)
- **The Soft Drink Industry** – #1 client for the sugar industry.
- **The Fast Food Industry** – Combines fat, salt and sugar in the right combinations to keep us returning for more hamburgers, fries and so

HOW VALID ARE SCIENTIFIC NUTRITION STUDIES?

Annually, there are approximately 100,000 nutrition studies carried out by different organizations, following different protocols and, frequently, with conflicting conclusions. The question is…How do we know which studies are valid and which are not? To establish whether or not a study is truly reliable or, in fact biased, we would need to know:

1) **Who authored the study?**
2) **Who sponsored the study?**
3) **What type of study was it (i.e., double blind, randomized, controlled, etc.)**

I doubt that most people, including myself, bother to investigate the studies sufficiently, in order to answer those questions. Since studies can and are often skewed either way, depending on the author, the sponsor or the type, we can simply pick and choose which ones support our beliefs and/or habits...or as Dr. John McDougall states, "We love to hear good things about our bad habits." Even Big Tobacco used studies that said nice things about smoking.

Seven years ago a close friend of mine, Beatriz from Cozumel, Mexico, went through open heart surgery, at the age of 72. Because of complications, one year later, she was told that she would need the insertion of a stent. However, the artery from her leg, that replaced the original one, turned out to be too narrow for the stent. The doctor told her that, unfortunately, there was nothing they could do...so they sent her home. She was given a few months to live. At the time I found out about her situation, I had already been following a Whole Food Plant Based diet (WFPB). I told her about several doctors and health care professionals that were having remarkable success with reversing heart disease with a WFPB diet. I also gave her the NY Times best seller, "Prevent and Reverse Heart Disease", by the Cleveland Clinic surgeon, Dr. Caldwell Esselstyn...the book responsible for changing Bill Clinton's life. Beatriz became inspired and, 7 years later (not 7 months) is doing very well and hasn't experienced another heart incident during these years. Although Beatriz's success is not included in any clinical study, what's obvious is that both of us have experienced the undeniable power of WFPB nutrition.

While powerful corporations and institutions manipulating scientific studies, there are increasing numbers of

Drs. and Health Care Practitioners, around the world who are curing their patients with Whole Plant Based foods and showing the extraordinary potential of a Whole Food Plant Based diet in Preventing and Reversing Heart Disease, Cancer, Type 2 Diabetes, Osteoporosis, Arthritis, etc. Just to name a few that I'm inspired by: *Dr. Caldwell Esselstyn, Dr. Michael Greger, Dr. John McDougall, Dr. Neal Bernard, Dr. Dean Ornish, Dr. John Robbins, Dr. E. Colin Campbell and Dr. Joel Fuhrman.* Maybe it's time for people to pay more attention to this type of one on one evidence, instead of relying so much on scientific studies that are often confusing, biased and questionable.

CAN NUTRITION STUDIES BE TRUSTED?
PART 2

Yesterday was a banner day for me as my Go Whole Food Vegan Facebook page reached 1000+ followers...all from this year. Today I checked the statistics and what jumped right out at me is that 1/3 of my page followers are between the ages of 18 – 24 and more than 50% between 18 and 34. What a pleasant surprise because it indicates to me that there's a lot more interest in our health and wellbeing among the youth, than I expected. I remember how I was, so I thought that young people would be more focused on their social lives, sports, education and their careers...than personal health. What a nice surprise to see that some things have changed. I thought that older people, would be more likely to follow my posts, because illness and disease would become a more prominent factor as we get older. Yet in the

65+ age group only 8% are following my page. I guess I was dead wrong on several things I imagined. Imagination will only take you so far.

Added note: *67% of those following my page are women.*

Now, to get back to the title of this post:

I have been having a wonderful and sometimes challenging time responding to people's comments to my posts. Last week I received several comments to my Can Nutrition Studies Be Trusted (Part 1) but one comment in particular, attracted my attention: Despite all the propaganda, there isn't any evidence that vegan diets are any better than other diets. To support this, he attached the following scientific study:

The Title: Mortality in Vegetarians and comparable Non-Vegetarians (including vegans), in the United Kingdom

The study was done in 2015 with the participation of 60,000+ persons, including approximately 40,000 meat and/or fish eaters, 18,096 vegetarians (dairy but no meat) and 2228 vegans who don't eat meat or dairy. The study was very complete, with comparative tables, footnotes and quite a few references.

So what, in this study, didn't sit right with me?

For those who have been following my posts, you know that when I refer to vegan nutrition I mean exclusively Whole Food Vegan or Whole Food Plant Based (WFPB) nutrition. That is why my Facebook page is titled, Go Whole Food Vegan. In other words, if the food is not whole food, then it's processed and/or refined, which could very well spell health problems, somewhere down the line, including chronic diseases.

Several months ago I published a post entitled "Not All Vegans Are Created Equal." What I explained is that there are 2 categories of vegans: 1) Persons with a primary interest in their personal health through a WFPB diet and 2) Ethical or Moral vegans who have a primary interest in the no exploitation or torture of animals as well as the saving of the Earth's environment. Generally, although they don't consume meat or dairy, eating whole foods is often not as much a priority as it is for the category 1 vegan. A couple of years ago I became aware of this difference when I joined an online vegan group that had more than 100,000 members. When someone asked the question, *"Is Coca Cola vegan?"*, there were many replies… some yeses and some nos. I then replied: *"What does it matter?*

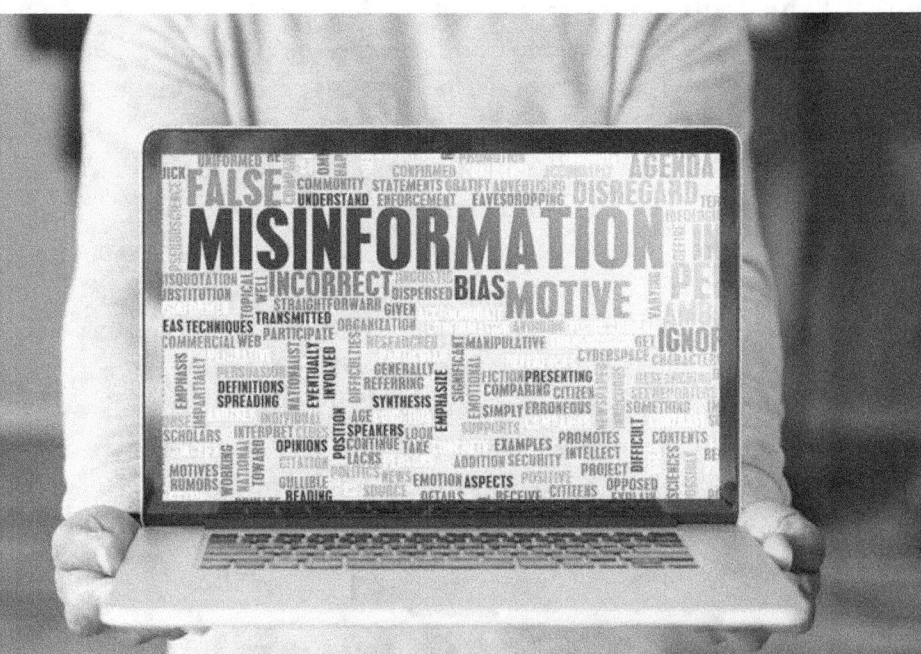

Coca Cola is not healthy!" I soon received an unexpected response from the groups creator, no less: "As a vegan, it doesn't matter what one eats… as long as it doesn't involve animal exploitation." With health as my priority, I left the group.

With regards to the above study, without revealing what the 2228 vegans were eating, how could we possibly know if they were consuming a healthy Whole Foods diet or not? On the contrary, their regular diet could have been based on fried potatoes, cakes, donuts and pastries, white bread, white rice, refined pasta and sugar, high fructose corn syrup, texturized soy etc… all washed down with a nice cold glass of coca cola. Yes, they're "officially" vegans, but the diet could very well be as unhealthy as people on the Standard American Diet of meat, dairy and processed and refined foods.

What was the conclusion from this study?
"Our results suggest that United Kingdom–based vegetarians and comparable non- vegetarians (including people who eat fish but not meat and those who eat meat <5 times per week on average) have similar all-cause mortality. The differences by diet group found for specific causes of death merit further investigation."

I don't understand why vegans and vegetarians were lumped together for this study. If the point is to compare diets in order to get accurate mortality results, it should be necessary to include Whole Food vegans as a separate group, not as a part of the vegetarian group, which consumes milk and dairy products. Vegans do not consume meat or dairy…and therefore, should be respected for that. Fact is that populations on a WFPB diet (*rural Japan and China, parts of rural Africa and the 5 Blue Zones – Okinawa, Japan, Ikaria, Greece, Sardinia, Italy, Nicoya, Costa Rica and Loma Linda, California*) not only live longer than people on the Standard American Diet, but rarely suffer the pain and premature death…from the same chronic diseases. Long term studies are also proving that the WFPB diet has the power to help prevent common illnesses and chronic diseases, by strengthening the body's immune system and clinical studies, carried out with their patients, by renowned Doctors (i.e., Drs. Caldwell Esselstyn, Michael Greger, John McDougall, Dean Ornish, Neal Barnard, Joel Fuhrman, T. Colin Campbell, Michael Klaper, Kim Williams, etc.), are consistently showing the disease reversal powers of WFPB nutrition, especially with regards to Heart Disease, Type 2 Diabetes, Certain Cancers, Osteoporosis, High Blood Pressure and Obesity.

6

HEALTH: PERSONAL, ANIMAL AND THE PLANET

"You cannot get through a single day without having an impact on the world around you. What you do makes a difference, and you have to decide what kind of difference you want to make."

Jane Goodall, author of 32 books on animals and the environment

CLIMATE CHANGE
PART 1
Is Carbon Dioxide Really the Main Problem?

For me, the experience of not consuming meat for more than 40 years and dairy for the past 8 years, combined with fact based nutrition research, has led me to conclude that Whole

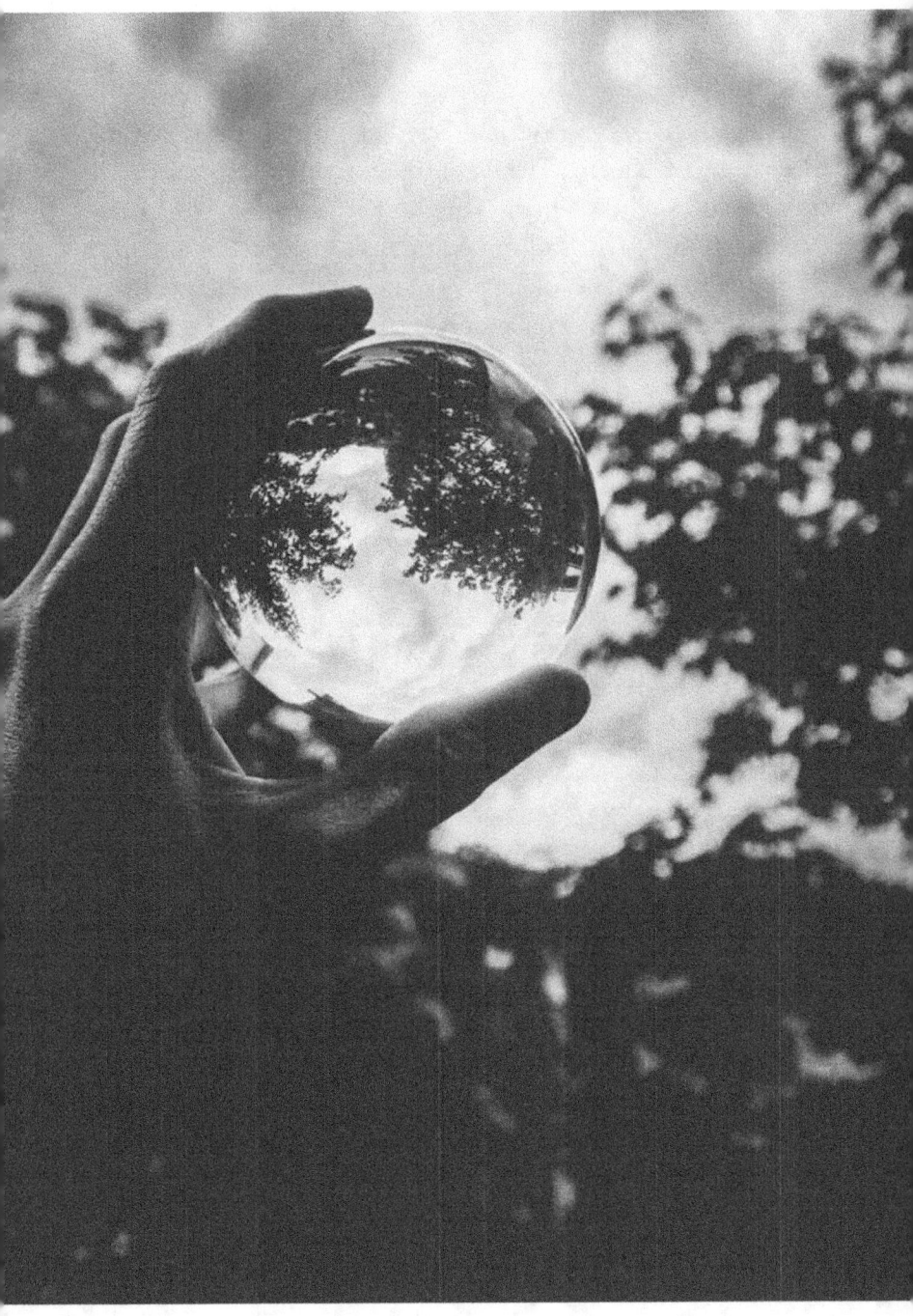

Food Plant Based nutrition is the healthiest path to optimal health and wellbeing. However, personal health is not the main reason why so many people are becoming vegetarians (no meat) or vegans (no meat or dairy). Instead, it's mainly a response to animal exploitation and cruelty as well as the devastating effects that climate change is having on our planet. For them, not consuming animal products, in any form, is the best way to reverse climate change.

The main objective of this two part series on Climate Change is to inform and explain how what we eat effects the Global Environment.

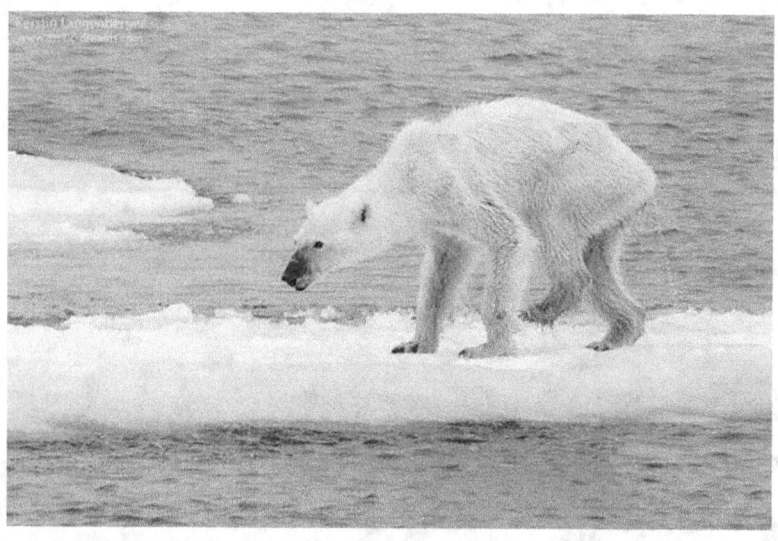

What are The Consequences of Climate Change?
According to the Third and Fourth National Climate Assessment Reports (NASA): *"Global climate change has*

already had observable effects on the environment. Glaciers have shrunk, ice on rivers and lakes is breaking up earlier, plant and animal ranges have shifted and trees are flowering sooner. Effects that scientists had predicted in the past would result from global climate change are now occurring: loss of sea ice, accelerated sea level rise and longer, more intense heat waves."

And The Future...

"Climate Change will continue through this century and beyond and the way things are going some of the long-term effects of global climate change we can expect are as follows:

- Temperatures will continue to rise
- Frost Free Season and Growing Season will lengthen
- More droughts and Heat Waves
- Hurricanes will become stronger and more intense
- Sea level will Rise 1 – 4 feet by 2100
- Arctic to become ice free by mid-century

Each of the past three decades has been warmer than any preceding decade since weather records began in 1850. Today, the world's leading climate scientists believe that human activities are almost certainly the main cause of the warming observed since the middle of the 20th century.

An increase of 2°C (3.6° F) compared to the temperature in preindustrial times is seen by scientists as the threshold beyond which there is a much higher risk that dangerous and possibly catastrophic changes in the global environment will occur. For this reason, in 2016 the international community of 200 countries came together in Paris and came up with the Paris Agreement which has, as it's main goal, the need to keep global warming below 2°C. In order to do this, there is a need to reduce gas emissions."

How does that work?

Some gases in the Earth's atmosphere act a bit like the glass in a greenhouse, trapping the sun's heat and stopping it from going back into space and although many of these gases occur naturally, human activity is increasing the concentrations of some of them in the atmosphere, in particular:

- **carbon dioxide (CO2)**
- **methane**
- **nitrous oxide**

According to the Paris Agreement these are the main Causes of the Rising of Gas Emissions:

- Burning of fossil fuels: coal, oil and gas which produces carbon dioxide and nitrous oxide.
- Cutting down rainforests (deforestation). Trees help to regulate the climate by absorbing CO2 from the atmosphere. So when they are cut down, that beneficial effect is lost and the carbon stored in the trees is released into the atmosphere, adding to the greenhouse effect.
- Increasing livestock farming. Cows and sheep produce large amounts of methane when they digest their food and release gas.

According to the Agreement, the burning of fossil fuels is by far the main culprit while the effects of methane gas is not considered that important. As a result, the responsibility of stopping and/or reversing the tendency towards global warming lies mainly in the hands of large industries, especially transportation, which depends on the burning of fossil fuels.

The question is...is Carbon Dioxide in the atmosphere the main cause of Global Warming?

It is, according to António Guterres, the United Nations secretary general. He told global leaders during a speech this month (September) at the U.N. headquarters in New York that the world has less than two years to avoid "runaway climate change." "The time has come for our leaders to show they care about the people whose fate they hold in their hands," Guterres said. "We need to rapidly shift away from our dependence on fossil fuels."

What about Methane and other Gases from Livestock?

According to a report, "Livestock's Long Shadow – Environmental Issues and Options", released in November of 2006 from the United Nations Food and Agriculture Organization,

"Livestock emerges as one of the top two or three most significant contributors to every one of the most serious environmental problems. The livestock sector is a major player, responsible for 18 percent of greenhouse gas emissions. This is a higher share than transport. (Note: The release of this report was not covered by any of the major news outlets, only a few mentions are found on the Internet).

So, which is it?

The dilemma we're in is that, if the problem is CO2, then the responsibility of turning Climate Change around lies mainly in the hands of industry. If the main problem is Methane and other gases...and the solution is actually connected to livestock...to a much greater extent the responsibility and the power of effecting change lies in the hands of each one of us.

In Part 2: The Solution is on Our Plate...I will explain how our choices can make a difference and how we, as citizens of Planet Earth, have the power to reverse Climate Change.

CLIMATE CHANGE
PART 2
The Solution is On Your Plate

I believe that most of us understand that what we eat effects our health, either positively or negatively, but I think that too few of us are aware of the effects that what we eat has on the Earth's environment...including it's animals, water, pollution and land damage. One of the problems is that, although 98% of the meat we eat comes from factory farms, we are very far removed from what is happening, behind the scenes, when we buy the packaged meat at the supermarket or from the local butcher shop. Whereas 50 years ago, a rancher would have 10 head of cattle, now factory farms handle thousands at a time.

The result is that the average person is so far removed from the realities of factory farms that they are unaware of the enormous damage they have on the Earth's environment...in the following areas:

Atmospheric Damage
Land Damage
Water Scarcity
Water Pollution
Destruction of Species

The United Nations Food and Agriculture Organization Report:

According to the report, "Livestock's Long Shadow —Environmental Issues and Options", released in November of 2006 from the United Nations Food and Agriculture Organization, livestock emerges as one of the top two or three most significant contributors to every one of the most serious environmental problems. With rising temperatures, rising sea levels, melting icecaps and glaciers, shifting ocean currents and weather patterns, climate change is the most serious challenge facing the human race. The livestock sector is a major player, responsible for 18 percent of greenhouse gas emissions. This is a higher share than transport which emits 13.5 percent. In addition to CO_2, environmentally toxic gases produced by livestock include nitrous oxide, methane, and ammonia generated from the animals' intestines—belching, farting, and manure. The report says "The impact is so severe that it needs to be addressed with urgency." (Note: The release of this report was not covered by any of the major news outlets, only a few mentions are found on the Internet).

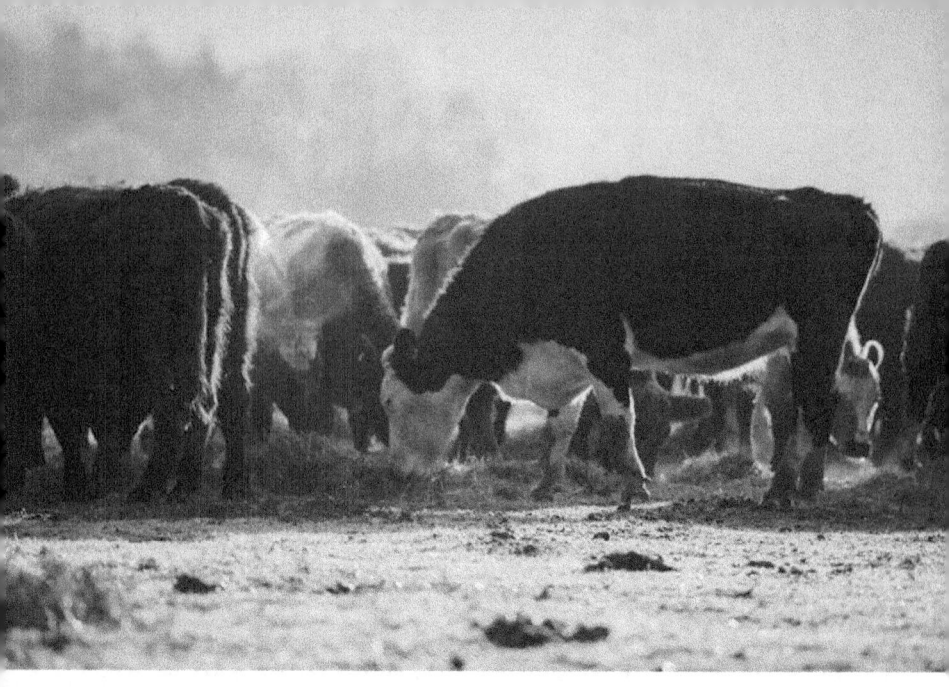

ATMOSPHERIC DAMAGE:

According to Dr. James Hansen, Director of NASA's Goddard Institute for Space Studies and who has been called *"a grandfather of the global warming theory"*:

"The focus solely on CO_2 is fueled in part by misconceptions. It's true that human activity produces vastly more CO_2 than all other greenhouse gases put together. However, this does not mean it is responsible for most of the earth's warming. Many other greenhouse gases trap heat far more powerfully than CO_2, some of them tens of thousands of times more powerfully. When taking into account various gases' global warming potential—defined as the amount of actual warming a gas will produce over the next one hundred years—it turns out that gases other than CO_2 (methane, nitrous oxide and ammonia) make up most of the global warming problem." Again, livestock is the main producer of these gases.

LAND DAMAGE:

- Globally, 70% of the total arable land is occupied by grazing livestock. Of the other 30%, 28% is for bio-fuel and only 2% for human consumption.
- Every 2 seconds, an area the size of a soccer field is destroyed in order to feed livestock, so that the world's need for meat can be satisfied. In other words, we're feeding animals instead of feeding people. Unfortunately, 1 billion people suffer from hunger and more than 30,000,000 die from hunger each year.
- According to the United Nations World Food Program it is estimated that a person dies of hunger or hunger-related causes every ten seconds. Sadly, it is children who die most often.
- Clearing forests to create new pastures is a major source of deforestation, especially in Latin America. 70% of the Amazon rainforests have been cut down for grazing land. These tropical forests are the "lungs of the Earth" and vital for removing greenhouse gases from the atmosphere.

WATER SCARCITY:

We've all heard about the scarcity of water around the world and some of us do our best to limit water use (i.e., shorter showers, watering the lawn less frequently, washing dishes with less water). We don't realize that there are roughly 100 million cows in North America alone that require enormous amounts of food. Without a steady supply of soy and corn, which by the way is not a cow's natural food, slaughter houses would grind to a halt and our demand for meat and dairy would not be met. As a result, millions of acres are devoted to feed crops instead of human consumption. These crops need more water than any other human activity. Most of the water comes from irrigation which results in a huge drain on the water supply. This is happening around the world.

Comparison of Water Requirements to Produce Certain Foods:

Animal based foods:
1 kilo of chicken requires 3900 liters of water 1 kilo of cheese requires 5000 liters of water 1 kilo of beef requires 15,500 liters of water Plant Based Foods:
1 kilo of grain requires 1300 liters of water
1 kilo of potatoes requires 900 liters of water 1 kilo of apples requires 700 liters of water

"Imagine how much water we could save and how many starving people could be fed if the arable land was used for feeding humans instead of animals."

WATER POLLUTION:

- **Livestock pollutes the waters with their waste, antibiotics, hormones, chemicals from tanneries, fertilizers and the pesticides used to spray the crops they consume. These toxic elements seep into the earth and end up in rivers and streams. As** an example, in the Gulf of Mexico, below Texas and Louisiana, there is an 8,000 square mile dead zone, caused by fertilizers entering the Mississippi River...from the planting of soy and corn all along the River...to feed animals.

• Each kilo of meat that is produced results in 6 kilos of livestock excrement. And where does this end up...in huge lagoons, where the anaerobic activity releases methane into the atmosphere and ammonia into the water which causes acid rain and acidification of ecosystems. In other words, while human waste is treated...animal waste is not. It's just piled higher and higher and deeper and deeper.

DESTRUCTION OF SPECIES:
According to the United Nations Report, livestock's very presence in vast tracts of land and its demand for feed crops also contribute to loss of other plants and animals; livestock is identified as a culprit in 15 out of 24 important global ecosystems that are in decline. The loss of species is estimated to be running 50 to 500 times higher than previous recorded rates. When rainforests are cut down, animals can no longer compete and are forced to flee. Those unable to adapt will not survive.

CONCLUSION:

The primary driver of climate change isn't plastics, or cars, or airplanes. It's actually our industrialized food

206 MICHAEL J. DORFMAN

system? Sometimes I think that we're being distracted when focus is put on eliminating plastic straws and bags in stores and supermarkets instead of focusing on eliminating the main cause. I'm not against any effort because every little bit counts but I believe we need to have more fact based information and clarity on the subject of Climate Change. Only then can we put our energy and resources where it really counts. While governments debate about vehicle and smoke-stack emissions and environmental groups complain that little is being done, the fact is that we can tackle the main problem by changing our eating habits. What we eat has by far the largest impact on climate change.

I'm not advocating that it's necessary to eat 100% vegan or even become a vegetarian. If what I have written, in these past 2 posts, makes sense to you then simply by choosing more environmentally friendly foods at meal-time every day (i.e., grains, vegetables, fruits, nuts and seeds) we can help reduce and even reverse the global warming problem. I believe that it's time for the citizens of the world to make a difference.

HOW CAN WE KILL 3 BIRDS WITH ONE STONE?

What impressed me from the responses to my last 2 articles on Climate Change were the hundreds of sad faces (emogis) that people posted. Yes, the situation is sad...but fortunately there's still time to change things around. This follow-up article shares the hope that I have...that together we can make a difference.

With regards to the title, don't get me wrong. I'm not interested in killing 3 birds with one stone…not even 1 bird with 1 stone. It's just to emphasize the power of this particular stone.

So, what are the 3 birds?

1. Climate Change
2. Factory Farms
3. Chronic Diseases

And…the Stone?

WHOLE FOOD PLANT BASED NUTRITION (WFPB)

So let's get started…

1·CLIMATE CHANGE:

There are a lot of Naysayers who either don't believe in Climate Change or Global Warming or do believe but think that it's a natural occurring cycle that has appeared during different

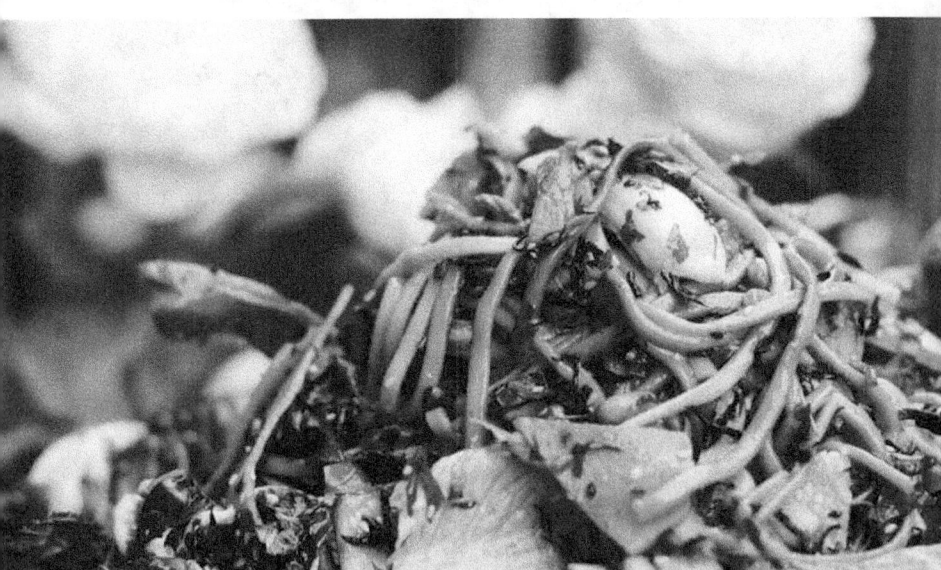

eras throughout the Earth's history and that human beings are not the cause and cannot change the course. My response to those people is *"Not only do 97% of scientists worldwide agree that climate change is happening at a faster rate than ever before but nearly 200 worldwide scientific organizations hold the position that this time climate change has been caused by human action."*

Maybe we're not at the point where we can say with 100% accuracy that humans are completely responsible for climate change, but if we accept the belief that humans have nothing to do with it, as some of the deniers claim, aren't we setting ourselves up for possible global catastrophes…maybe 50 or 100 years in the future? However, if the opposite is true…that humans are to blame…then maybe, if we "put our noses to the grindstone" we can come up with the necessary solutions.

Statement on climate change from 18 scientific associations:

> *"Observations throughout the world make it clear that climate change is occurring, and rigorous scientific research demonstrates that the greenhouse gases emitted by human activities are the primary driver."*

If we combine that statement with the information on greenhouse gases that I presented in my last 2 posts (methane, nitrous oxide and carbon dioxide), and begin to substitute grains, vegetables, fruits, nuts and seeds for animal products (meat, dairy and eggs), we can begin to slow down and eventually stop the emissions of greenhouse gases into the atmosphere.

2·FACTORY FARMS:

Factory farming is the intensive confinement of farmed animals raised for food and invented during the 1950s and 60s by scientists who knew that there was no way to continue feeding animal products to an increasing human population...without a significant increase in efficiency. Allowing animals, such as cows, chickens and pigs to roam free required vast expanses of land and was no longer feasible to satisfy the billions of meat eaters around the world. Grass-fed animals also require more food because the animals gain weight slower on a grass diet than they do with a manufactured, concentrated feed, which is most often not the natural food of these animals.

As I pointed out in my last 2 posts (Climate Change – The Solution is on Your Plate), the methane and nitrous oxide gas emissions from factory farm animals are the number 1 cause of global warming. This is supported by the United Nations Food and Agricultural Organization:

"The livestock sector is a major player, responsible for 18 percent of greenhouse gas emissions. This is a higher share than transport which emits 13.5 percent. In addition to CO2, environmentally toxic gases produced by livestock include nitrous oxide, methane, and ammonia generated from the animals' intestines—belching, farting, and manure. The report says "The impact is so severe that it needs to be addressed with urgency."

Hence, the only way factory farms, with the inhumane treatment of animals, can be abolished is by the reduction of the demand for meat and that will only happen if:

- The public becomes aware of the horrible environment and inhumane treatment and torture that factory farm animals experience.
- People stop seeing farm animals as commercial products and begin to see that, just like our pet dogs and cats, they have feelings too.
- The truth about the healthier protein from plants becomes widely accepted, especially by doctors and other health practitioners.
- People begin to accept the facts regarding the effect that factory farms are having on climate change.

3·CHRONIC DISEASE:

It is now well known that diet plays a huge factor in preventing and fighting chronic diseases, yet many healthcare providers, including our own doctors, are unaware of this research. These are the doctors we go to and trust as the ultimate health experts, yet they are missing vital information on how we can prevent disease in the first place. Initially, it's not their fault and they're doing the best they know how to do. Unfortunately, very few medical schools dedicate more than a few hours on nutrition, during a doctor's education. Their training is mainly focused on treating the symptoms of illness and disease, through pharmaceutical medicines and interventions such as chemotherapy, surgery and radiation. When it comes to diet, yes they may say "It's important to lose weight, cut down on saturated fats and lower cholesterol but in most cases that's about how specific it gets.

This just gets me thinking about how important it is for us to educate ourselves on everything that is out there… from conventional treatments to integrative and lifestyle approaches… and then make an educated decision on our own path to health. It just makes sense that the better that we treat our body and mind through lifestyle choices such as whole food plant based nutrition, exercise, stress avoidance and environmental factors, the healthier we will be.

How do we know this? Well, in populations that follow these choices (rural China, Japan, parts of Africa and the Blue Zones), people live longer and the illnesses and chronic diseases that we suffer and die from (i.e., heart disease, cancer, type 2 diabetes, osteoporosis, obesity, high blood pressure, etc.), are almost non-existent there.

The Good News is that…
Since a Whole Food Plant Based diet is that one stone that can tackle Climate Change, Factory Farms and Chronic Diseases head on, it's a great solution all around…a win- win situation for people, animals and the planet. What makes this so promising and gives us hope is that the solution doesn't lie in the hands of big businesses or the government. It lies in the hands of each human being and because of that…we have the power of choice to make the difference.

RECOMMENDED RESOURCES

RECOMMENDED RESOURCES

Since learning and discovery is a lifelong process, I would like to suggest the following books, cookbooks, websites and documentaries that have helped and inspired me to write this book and to "keep on trucking" along the path towards optimal health and nutrition.

Books on Health and Nutrition
— a few that have inspired me - * contain recipes
T. Colin Campbell, PhD and Thomas M. Campbell II, MD, The China Study — Revised Edition (Dallas, TX: BenBella Books, 2016)
T. Colin Campbell, PhD with Howard Jacobson, PhD, Whole — (Dallas, TX: Ben Bella Books, 2014)
Dr. Caldwell Esselstyn, Prevent and Reverse Heart Disease (New York: Avery, 20079)* Dr. Michael Greger, How Not to Die (New York: Flatiron Books, 2015)

Dr. John A. McDougall and Mary McDougall, The Starch Solution (Emmaus, PA: Rodale, 2012)* Dr. Dean Ornish, The Spectrum (New York: Ballantine Books, 2007)*
Dr. Dean Ornish, UnDo It! (New York: Ballantine Books, 2019)*
Dr. Neal Barnard, The Cheese Trap (New York: Grand Central Publishing, 2017)* Dr. Neal Barnard, Program for Reversing Diabetes (Emmaus, PA: Rodale, 2018) Dr. Joel Fuhrman, Eat to Live (New York, Little, Brown and Co., 2011)
Dr. David L. Katz, The Truth About Food (New York, Dystel and Goderich, 2018)* Ocean Robbins, 31 Day Food Revolution (New York: Grand Central Publishing, 2019)*

Cookbooks
Dr. Michael Greger, The How Not to Die Cookbook (New York: Flatiron Books, 2017)
Dr. Rip Esselstyn and Jane Esselstyn, The Engine 2 Cookbook (New York: Grand Central Publishing, 2017)
Cathy Fisher, Straight Up Food (Santa Rosa, Ca: Green Bite Publishing, 2016)
Lindsay Nixon, The Happy Herbivore Cookbook (Dallas, TX: Ben Bella Books, 2011) Dreena Burton, Plant Powered Families (Dallas, TX: Ben Bella Books, 2015)
Del Sroufe, Forks Over Knives – The Cookbook (New York: Experiment, 2012)
Alan Roettinger, Extraordinary Vegan (Summertown, TN: Book Publishing Co., 2013) Leanne Campbell, The China Study Cookbook (Dallas, TX: Ben Bella Books, 2013)

Websites for Information and Recipes

NutritionFacts.org brings you Dr. Michael Greger's fact based research through daily videos and posts on just about every nutrition subject. It's my favorite site for fact base research.

Forks Over Knives (forks overknives.com) has great recipes, meal planning, success stories and more.

Dr. McDougall's Health and Medical Center (drmcdougall. com) Lots of information on his starched based diet, recipes from his wife Mary and free bi-monthly livestream interviews with doctors and nutrition experts.

Physicians Committee for Responsible Medicine (pcrm.org) features a 21 Day Vegan Kickstart program, latest nutrition information and recipes.

Center for Nutrition Studies (nutritionstudies.org) from T. Colin Campbell, author of the International Best Seller, "The China Study", includes information on a wide variety of health topics as well as recipes.

Isa Chandra (isachandra.com) has a practical ingredient-based recipe finder.

Pinterest (pinterest.com) allows you to search for and sav vegan recipes while offering new ones the next time you visit.

Plant-Based on a Budget (plantbasedonabudget.com) teaches you how to make healthy and economical vegan meals.

Vegetarian Resource Group (vrg.org) great information from expert writers that supports a vegan lifestyle.

Note: These are only a few of the websites that offer vegan recipes

Documentaries

<u>Forks Over Knives</u> is a ground breaking documentary with interviews of doctors and experts in the field of nutrition. Can be seen on Netflix as well as on youtube.

<u>What the Health</u> confronts established institutions that have been misleading the public with regards to our health and disease. Available on Netflix and youtube.

<u>H.O.P.E. What You Eat Matters</u> has won many awards. Shows the relationship between what we eat and our personal health, the health of the planet and the exploitation of animals. Available on Netflix and youtube.

<u>Plant Pure Nation</u> pulls the curtain back on the corporate interests behind the food industry and how that influences laws and social norms. Includes interviews with doctors and experts. Available on Amazon.

<u>Cowspiracy</u> exposes the exploitation and deplorable treatment of animals on "factory farms." Available on Netflix and youtube.